gua sha
& crystal
massage

gua sha & crystal massage

Techniques for Healthy,
Clear, and Glowing Skin

JULIE CIVIELLO POLIER

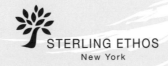

STERLING ETHOS
New York

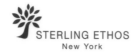

STERLING ETHOS
New York

An Imprint of Sterling Publishing Co., Inc.

ISBN 978-1-4549-4844-5
ISBN 978-1-4549-4845-2 (ebook)

Distributed in Canada by Sterling Publishing Co., Inc. c/o Canadian Manda
Group, 664 Annette Street, Toronto, Ontario M6S 2C8, Canada

For information about custom editions, special sales, and premium
purchases, please contact specialsaes@unionsquareandco.com.

Printed in China

unionsquareandco.com

Conceived, designed, and produced by Quarto Publishing plc
an imprint of The Quarto Group
The Old Brewery,
6 Blundell Street
London N7 9BH
www.quarto.com

QUAR.355838

2 4 6 8 10 9 7 5 3 1

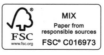

MIX
Paper from
responsible sources
FSC® C016973

FSC
www.fsc.org

Caution

Contents

Meet Julie

Gua sha found me. I fondly think of our introduction in this way. An elegant jade facial roller caught my eye in a facial treatment room around the time I was finishing aesthetician school. The roller leaped off the shelf toward me completely unprompted. This tool piqued my interest, setting me off on a deep-dive exploration of many techniques until I surfaced in the traditional practices of gua sha.

It all started with my mother, who sought out the healing support of acupuncture during her pregnancy with me because she had heard about the "beautiful baby point" that is only used with a 24-karat gold needle. When I was old enough to receive the needles myself, my mom took me with her to mother and daughter acupuncture practitioners Fern and Maureen Tsao, in Yarmouth, Maine. I received a transformational education with these acupuncturists that opened up a world of healing I had never thought possible before. I am so grateful to my mother for introducing me to healing methods that, at the time, were considered wildly alternative, yet we knew them to be incredibly effective. And 31 years after receiving the golden needle in utero, I too offered the "beautiful baby point" to our son while carrying him.

After considering career paths that included film and acupuncture, I chose facial massage because I have a leaning toward the gentlest modality for alchemy. I have seen the greatest transformations occur from the most tender of touches. Also, facial massage is easily taught, and another great love of mine is to share my wisdom, to expand yours and another's own innate healing abilities.

It is with great joy that I have created this book for you, and it is my intention that you, dear reader and masseuse, create many tender moments with yourself. I have found that massaging my face has been, and continues to be, my return to center, a way to harmonize all my bodies at once: the physical, the emotional, the mental, and the spiritual.

Curious where to start? A lot of people are. The truth is, you cannot do anything wrong. You will not ruin your face simply by intuitively and gently moving a tool around on your skin. Inviting these beautiful massages and gua sha practices into your beauty rituals is easiest when you keep it gentle, short, and sweet. Aim for light pressure, and follow what feels good. A little bit, consistently, goes a long way, but you do not have to practice daily—keep it fun and doable. I keep tools in my purse, car console, and coat pocket so that, wherever I am, I can fit in a few strokes to release jaw tension, or melt some thoughts by smoothing out my forehead.

May you benefit from this book by expanding your own practice of tuning into your body, learning more and more about the language you share with all your organs, and softening into the radiant beauty that is you and only you.

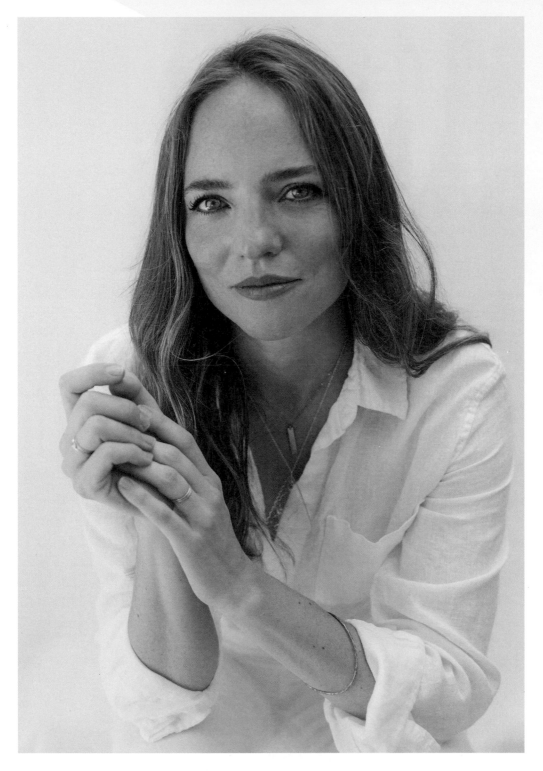

How to Navigate Through This Book

There is no right or wrong way to explore this book, my only wish is that it may serve you very well. You can read Chapters 1-3 (pages 10-47) first for an introduction to the practice of gua sha to learn more about how it works, or you can skip straight to Chapter 4 (pages 48-99) and start to massage right away.

There are step-by-step illustrations for each massage—these were all drawn from photographs and videos of me massaging my own face—so every routine is easy to follow, even for beginners.

If you want to know more about acupressure points and how you can use them in conjunction with gua sha massage, turn to Chapter 5 (pages 100-115). You will find Cool Down Routines in Chapter 6 (pages 116-129) which offer the added benefit of calm and restful sleep, and turn to Chapter 7 (pages 130-139) for Your Bespoke Treatment Plan, where you can find combined techniques for assisting with specific skin concerns.

KEY TO SYMBOLS

How long a massage will take

How many times to repeat a sequence

Which gua sha tool to use

The angle to hold the tool

How much pressure to apply

Which energy meridians we come into contact with

Which organs can benefit

Acupressure point location, only for pages 106–115

Caution—make sure you pay close attention to these notes, as they are important for your health and wellbeing

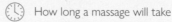

Quick Start Guide

Here are some short cuts if you'd like to address a "skin message," (see page 16) or you can also flip the book open to any page, which usually offers an instinctive, perfect remedy for that particular moment.

If you don't have much time...
* 1-Minute Facelift, *page 138*

To smooth wrinkles...
* Comb Edge Massage, *page 56*
* Lip Lines & Wrinkles, *page 60*
* Cheekbone Sculpt, *page 66*
* Crow's Feet Wrinkle Eraser, *page 80*
* Smoothing 11s Wrinkles, *page 90*
* Smoothing Horizontal Forehead Lines, *page 92*

To clear acne and blemishes...
* Terminus Tug, *page 41*
* Horseshoe Press, *page 43*
* Downward Neck Sweep, *page 50*
* Facial Beauty, *page 108*
* The Four Whites, *page 109*
* Joyful Sleep, *page 111*

To soften pigmentation...
* Comb Edge Massage, *page 56*
* Lip Lines & Wrinkles, *page 60*
* Fading Pigmentation Spots, *page 136*

To improve your skin's elasticity...
* Upward Neck Sweep, *page 54*
* Face Lift, *page 76*
* Third Eye Opener, *page 94*

To relieve dark circles or puffy eyes...
* Under-Eye Sweep, *page 78*
* Eye Press, *page 82*
* Thymus Press, *page 114*

In order to understand why and how gua sha massage works, it is beneficial to know more about its origins in traditional Chinese medicine (TCM), and how the techniques overlap with reflexology, the lymphatic system, and our energy meridians. This chapter seeks to provide a brief introduction to all these ancient practices.

Gua Sha Basics

CHAPTER 1

What is Gua Sha?

Hailing from Southeast Asia, gua sha is a traditional Chinese medicine practice in which various tools are applied to a person's skin. Like much traditional Chinese medicine, the exact origins of gua sha are unknown. The practice was first recorded nearly 700 years ago during the Ming dynasty (1368–1644), but oral traditions of the practice will have passed through many generations before that time, meaning that it likely has a much longer history.

Pronounced "gwah shah" or "gwah saw," in Chinese gua means "to scrape" and sha means "sand." Originally, the scraping was applied to the body rather than the face. Using a specific tool (see page 27), the practitioner made a series of strokes aimed at producing "petechiae"—visible red to purple bruising on the skin. The action was understood to release toxins from the circulatory system, bringing them to the surface of the skin, eliminating congestion in the process and increasing the flow of energy or "qi" (see page 15). The darker the bruising, the higher the concentration of toxic buildup. The practitioner followed the bruising, scraping deeper into the darker, purple areas while avoiding those that were lighter and pinker. Patterns developed, making the once invisible energy stagnation very visible in deep-purple lines usually across the back, neck, and shoulders. The practice remains little changed today.

Facial gua sha is much more gentle than body gua sha and uses very light pressure, so it does not cause any bruising. It is currently trending in the West and has become popular on social media platforms across the globe. The most common uses today are less concerned with holistic health and focus more on "anti-aging" and noninvasive face lifting. Even in these cases, however, one still receives all of the deeper benefits of the treatment, which includes tending to the vital organs, honoring the emotional body, and aligning all aspects of the self—even if one does not realize it. There are a few practitioners with large audiences who raise greater awareness of the deeper layers of this practice and honor its lineage and history. See Resources on page 141 for further exploration.

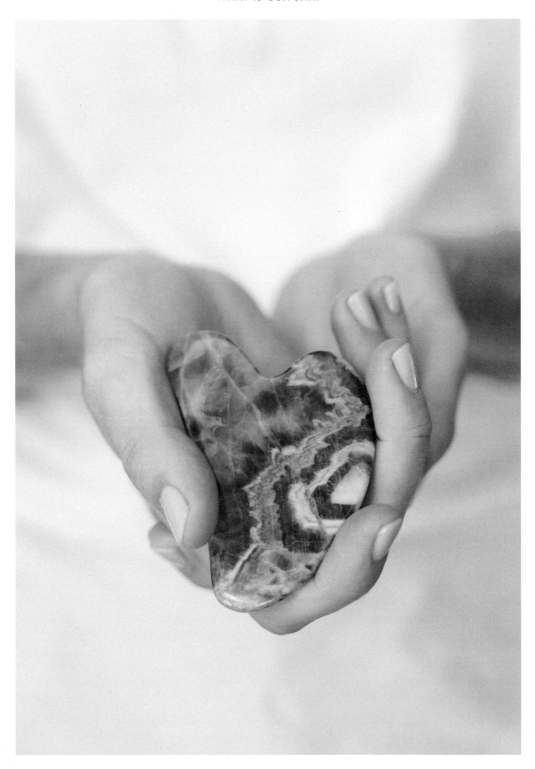

Traditional Chinese Medicine: the Roots of Gua Sha

Gua sha is one practice within traditional Chinese medicine (TCM), a multifaceted healing system born from alchemical Taoist texts and ancestral philosophy. Heavily documented in the *Tao Te Ching* written by Lao Tzu, TCM deeply honors the energy of "that which cannot be named," as acupuncturist Katya Mosely explains. The definitions in TCM can be very fluid, changing seasonally and dancing more in the vague and inclusive than in the exact and dissected. Even before Taoist alchemy, there were earlier traditions such as those of the Wu, Neolithic priests who functioned as healers rather than preachers. Wu was once one of the three great religions of China along with Buddhism and Confucianism.

Today, those of us who identify as Westerners may think of medical acupuncture or herbal supplementation when we think of TCM, but a truly holistic approach involves all aspects of a person's lifestyle, including diet, movement, meditation, breathwork, the interconnectedness of the body's systems with the energy bodies, moxibustion (burning dried mugwort herbs over acupressure points for relief), the use of herbal remedies, muscle testing, massage, and gua sha. In short, TCM and its philosophy treat body, mind, and spirit as one when it comes to healing.

For the purposes of this book, several other TCM practices are discussed alongside gua sha, in order to demonstrate their interconnectedness and to put the gua sha practice into context. They are energy meridians, acupressure, the concepts of yin and yang, the four bodies, the third eye, and reflexology. There are many more practices beyond this, so feel free to explore more if you wish.

The energy meridians are energetic pathways that run deep within the body, passing through each organ and muscle group. For a map of the body's meridians, see page 21.

Reflexology is a massage practice based on the concept that the anatomy of the body is reflected in miniature on areas of the face, hands, feet, and ears. It is closely connected to the energy meridians. For a reflexology map of the face, see page 17.

Acupressure points live along the meridian lines on the skin's surface and are pools of heat and electricity. Pressing on these points stimulates or redistributes the energy within the associated organ or system as well as the entire energetic meridian line itself. See pages 104-105 for a more in depth explanation and illustrations for how to find and work with your acupressure points.

Yin and yang are two complementary energies that create a whole, depicted as the black and white swirls that create a circle. Each swirl has a dot within, signifying the masculine and feminine energies within us all, always intending for equity and harmony. Typical yin traits and associations are: female, soft, passive, night, earth element, damp, cold, slow. Typical yang traits and associations are: male, hard, active, day, fire element, dry, heat, quick.

The four bodies is a concept in TCM that considers our physical, emotional, mental, and spiritual aspects to be equal and without separation. Like yin and yang, the four bodies are meant to be in harmony with each other, each maintaining one quarter of a human's experience.

Qi or "chi" in TCM often translates to "vital life force energy" and the Chinese character is two symbols together: the symbol for air and the symbol for rice, as culturally rice is thought of as a vital food that offers nourishment and sustenance. Qi translates to "air" or "breath" in the Chinese language.

The third eye originates in Hinduism, and is part of the chakra system that originated in the Indian Vedic scriptures as early as 500 BCE. Physiologically, the third eye correlates to the pineal gland, which French philosopher and author, René Descartes coined "the seat of the soul." The pineal gland supports reproductive hormones and assists the body to maintain with the circadian rhythm, waking with the dawn and resting by dusk. It brings great harmony to all aspects of the body and the four bodies.

EMOTIONAL HEALTH

Though TCM usually centers on our main aspects as spirit, body, and mind, I believe most, if not all, of our physical ailments have a root cause in the emotional and mental bodies. Our thoughts and emotions can dictate to the body how to function as well as throw off the body's inherent systems. Repeated thoughts and emotions create muscle memory and patterns in the body's fascia, the collagen matrix just under the skin.

Reflexology

Reflexology is the concept and associated massage practice that the entire anatomy of the body is reflected in miniature on reflex zones on the face (as well as the feet, hands, and ears). As such, it is closely connected to the meridian system (see pages 20-23).

In TCM, the organs and emotions have a bidirectional relationship. This means that an emotion associated with a given organ affects that organ, usually by throwing it off balance; similarly, the state and health of that organ affects the emotion. For example, the lungs are associated with grief. A person experiencing deep loss may also experience a lung infection, pneumonia, or develop a cough. This is understood as the body's way of purging and moving through the many layered emotions.

In Eastern philosophy and TCM it is practiced that the emotional life is understood through the body—its organs and systems—rather than understanding feelings through the psyche in the way Westerners categorize and analyze. *The Huangdi Neijing* (*The Yellow Emperor's Classic of Medicine*) is an ancient text exploring health through the TCM lens and is said to have been written by the Chinese emperor Huangdi around 2600 BCE. This book is one of the first to record emotions as having relationships with the organs.

Facial Organ Map
This map uses several facial reflexology charts from different lineages and practices. Having worked on so many faces in the facial treatment room, I developed this map to provide insight when "skin messages" may feel very complicated to unpack. Whenever a "skin message" pops up (psoriasis, hyperpigmentation, pimples, a new wrinkle), you can use this map to help identify which organ-emotion is in need of a balancing action and tailor your gua sha massage to address any issues that come up.

THE ORGAN–EMOTION CORRELATION	
ORGANS	EMOTIONS
lungs	grief
liver, gallbladder	anger, regret
kidneys	fear
heart	joy
spleen, pancreas, stomach	worry, overthinking, disgust

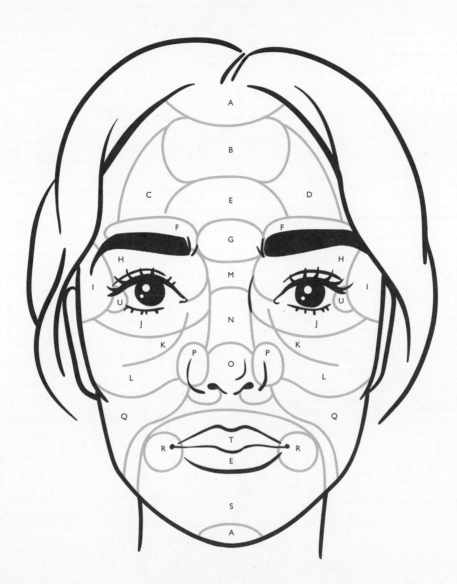

A: Bladder

B: Transverse colon

C: Ascending colon

D: Descending colon

E: Small Intestine

F: Fallopian tube

G: Liver

H: Gallbladder

I: Spleen

J: Kidney

K: Adrenal line

L: Large intestine

M: Pancreas

N: Spine

O: Heart + sex organs

P: Bronchi

Q: Lung

R: Duodenum

S: Sex hormones

T: Stomach

U: Ovaries/testes (entire eyes)

The Lymphatic System

In the body, in TCM, the circulatory system is considered to be yang/masculine and has the heart at its center: pulsing, nourishing, and fortifying blood to all parts of the body. The lymph is considered yin/feminine and does not have a pump. Instead, the lymph relies solely on movement, breathing, and loving massage to fortify the immune system by cleansing. Lymph is a watery fluid, clear to white in color, responsible for carrying toxins to the nearest lymph nodes, which cleanse and take care of the "trash," so to speak (see pages 38-47). Whenever your muscles are knotted and filled with tension, the fluids' pathways become restricted. This makes it more difficult for the blood to bring nutrients to each cell and obstructs the lymph from getting rid of waste.

While everyone is different, you have roughly 700 lymph nodes in your body and around one third of these are in your neck, just below the earlobes. The lymph nodes in your neck may swell when your body is fighting infection. This is often the first sign that your immune system is jumping into action. Gently massaging your neck using the techniques in this book are beneficial adjustments that open up the fluid pathways, allowing the fluids to do their jobs with ease.

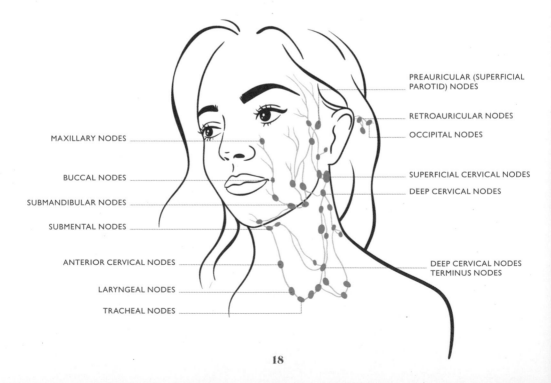

MAXILLARY NODES

BUCCAL NODES

SUBMANDIBULAR NODES

SUBMENTAL NODES

ANTERIOR CERVICAL NODES

LARYNGEAL NODES

TRACHEAL NODES

PREAURICULAR (SUPERFICIAL PAROTID) NODES

RETROAURICULAR NODES

OCCIPITAL NODES

SUPERFICIAL CERVICAL NODES

DEEP CERVICAL NODES

DEEP CERVICAL NODES
TERMINUS NODES

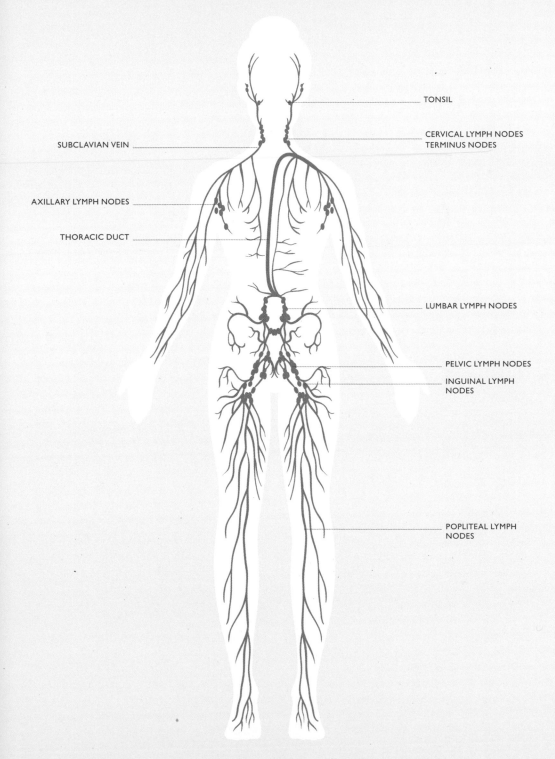

TONSIL

CERVICAL LYMPH NODES
TERMINUS NODES

SUBCLAVIAN VEIN

AXILLARY LYMPH NODES

THORACIC DUCT

LUMBAR LYMPH NODES

PELVIC LYMPH NODES

INGUINAL LYMPH
NODES

POPLITEAL LYMPH
NODES

The Energy Meridians

Communicating with the lymphatic fluids in the body, are the meridians. These energetic pathways support all the systems and organs of the body. Each runs through the neck, and using gua sha massage can be powerfully harmonizing, much like pressing an energetic reset button.

The conception vessel, sometimes called the central or ren meridian, offers energy to the uterus and genital organs, manages all of the yin/feminine channels and organs, supports creative developments, and assists with fertility, conception, pregnancy, and childbirth. The conception vessel receives qi, or life force energy, from all the yin meridians and then distributes this energy to the yang meridians.

The governing vessel guides all yang meridians and is associated with the immune system, energetically protecting the body from toxins and disease. The governing vessel is also considered to be the "fire" of the body, meaning it is responsible for the body's heat and vitality.

The triple warmer meridian is related to all the organs that regulate water in the body: lung, spleen, kidneys, small intestine, and bladder. This meridian might be considered "the nervous system meridian," operating our fight, flight, or freeze reactions and is yang/masculine. Since the nervous system propels the immune system, the triple warmer also has authority to activate immune responses. Deep breathing can be a great way to balance the triple warmer.

The stomach meridian is yang/masculine and manages the stomach, digestion; emotionally it relates to feelings of disgust and satiation.

The large intestine meridian is yang/masculine and manages the large intestine, the body's ability to eliminate waste, and how the body creates phlegm and mucus as a helpful means of disposal. Emotionally the large intestine is commonly associated with grief, however I personally find it is associated with "letting go" and often witness grief during this process.

The heart meridian is referred to in TCM as the "King of Organs," even though it is yin/feminine. It is the house of vital essence. Responsible for circulation and maintaining harmony in the emotions and thoughts, the heart meridian can reveal imbalances if the complexion is ashen or pallid. Any imbalance with the heart meridian will reverberate in imbalances throughout all other organs.

The pericardium meridian runs along the tissue that forms a protective sack around the heart. The pericardium meridian assists the heart and the triple warmer meridians with blood circulation as well as being the integrative layer between the emotional body and physical body in love making.

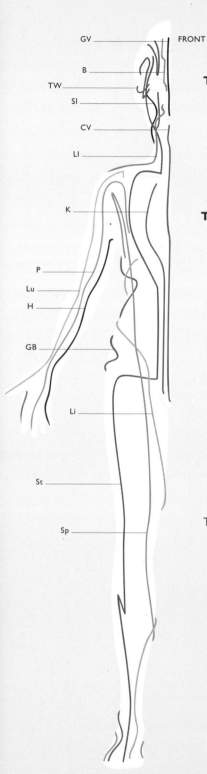
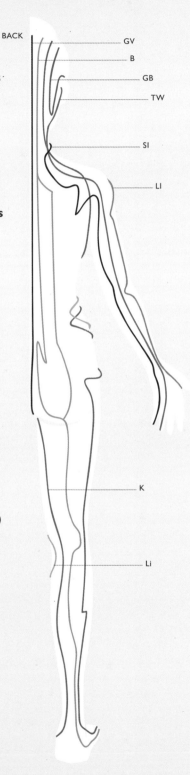

FRONT

BACK

GV

B

TW

SI

CV

LI

K

P

Lu

H

GB

Li

St

Sp

GV

B

GB

TW

SI

LI

K

Li

Two Centerline Meridians

● Governing Vessel (GV)

● Conception Vessel (CV)

Twelve Principal Meridians

● Stomach Meridian (St)

● Spleen Meridian (Sp)

● Small Intestine Meridian (SI)

● Heart Meridian (H)

● Bladder Meridian (B)

● Kidney Meridian (K)

● Pericardium Meridian (P)

● Triple Warmer Meridian (TW)

● Gallbladder Meridian (GB)

● Liver Meridian (Li)

● Lung Meridian (Lu)

● Large Intestine Meridian (LI)

The **kidney meridian** is yin/feminine and is the store of prenatal and vital energies. It is known as the "minister of power" as well as the "root of life."

The **spleen meridian** is referred to in TCM as the "minister of the granary," the yin/feminine spleen meridian includes the pancreas and assists with the extraction of nutrients because the spleen and pancreas generate enzymes to break down the food received by the stomach. This meridian also manages the quantity and quality of the blood. Like the kidney meridian, the spleen meridian aids in the formation of memory and plays a role in analytical thinking.

The **bladder meridian** is yang/masculine and is physically responsible for gathering and eliminating fluid waste. On an energetic level, it balances the autonomic nervous system, regulating the sympathetic and parasympathetic responses.

The **gallbladder meridian** is yang/masculine and secretes bile, aiding digestion and muscular energy. It is closely linked with the lymphatic system, since it is a member of the excretory organs. Emotionally, the gallbladder boosts our bold and risk-taking sensibilities.

The **small intestine meridian** is known as the "minister of reception," receives food during digestion, and is discerning in emotional nature, while physically separating the pure from the impure. Imbalances in the small intestine meridian can manifest as an inability to discern, a restlessness, a lack of reasoning and, physically, as digestion issues or emaciation on some level.

The **liver meridian** is yin/feminine and alchemizes nutrients from food into cellular plasma that translates to the rest of the body as energy and fuel. The liver also detoxifies the blood and assists the lymph as it is among the primary excretory organs. The liver meridian guides the peripheral nervous system and ligaments and tendons, so an inability to relax can indicate a liver imbalance. Challenges processing anger and rage are also an indication the liver may need support to balance once again.

The **lung meridian** works closely with the heart meridian to equalize energy and blood circulation throughout the body and is yin/feminine. The lung meridian generates radiant energy, strengthening the energetic field around the body, which both supports the immune system and the skin's vitality. Imbalances in the lungs can create skin issues, inflammation, breathing challenges or dysfunction, and imbalances in the emotions such as an excess of despair and anxiety.

Meridian lines on the head and neck

- Governing Vessel (GV)

- Conception Vessel (CV)

- Stomach Meridian (St)

- Small Intestine Meridian (SI)

- Bladder Meridian (B)

- Triple Warmer Meridian (TW)

- Gallbladder Meridian (GB)

- Large Intestine Meridian (LI)

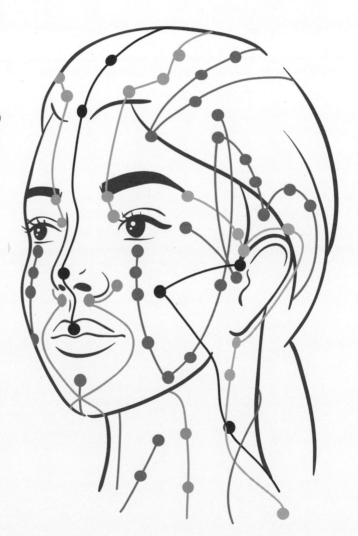

The gua sha tools of today come in a huge variety of shapes and materials, a selection of which are introduced in this chapter. The beauty and functionality of each tool and their particular uses help to create a sense of purpose and ritual in a self-care routine.

Gua Sha Tools

CHAPTER 2

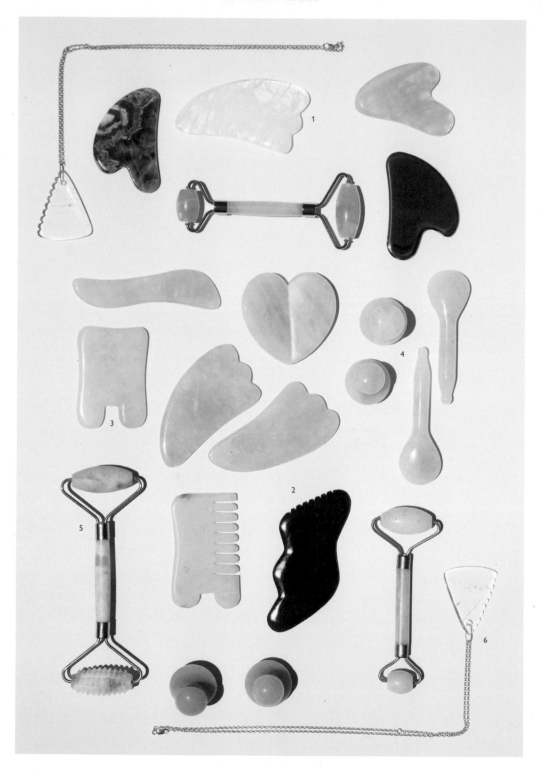

Basic Tools

In ancient times, gua sha tools were recycled materials or had a double purpose: coins, soup spoons, animal bones, cattle horns, and stones. Today, facial gua sha tools are typically made from polished and shaped crystals, which come in a wide range of shapes and sizes. Stainless-steel tools are also becoming increasingly popular, as this metal does not tarnish on the skin as brass and copper do.

Basic gua sha tool The simple wing or fin shape of this tool makes it ideal for many techniques. It has a slimmer point that fits well around the eyes and can efficiently contour under the cheekbones. (1)

Gua sha tool with notched edge A notch in the edge of a gua sha tool can be used to collect the tissue and guide more fascia and fluids in a given direction. This notch will gently grip the skin, whereas a smooth edge glides on top of the skin.

Gua sha tool with toothed edge Use the teeth to break up and smooth out wrinkles, scar tissue, or raised scar tissue called keloids. (2)

Gua sha tool with points or legs Use a tool with points or legs for tracing up either side of the back of the neck (hugging the spine) or tracing up the front of the neck (hugging the larynx). The edges of the points or legs are also effective for applying gentle pressure over acupressure points. (3)

Spoons or mushrooms Use a spoon or mushroom tool for massage and for tracing over the traditional gua sha patterns. A spoon/mushroom has less surface area and rounded edges, so is less useful for defining and contouring. (4)

Face roller Use a roller for massage and easing tension in tissues and muscles. A roller does not work as well as traditional gua sha massage tools. (5)

Gua sha tool on a necklace Having a tool to adorn yourself with makes it easy to massage anywhere and anytime because it is always with you. (6)

FIND WHAT SUITS YOU BEST

Facial tools seem to come in any size and shape imaginable. Keep turning your tool upside down and flipping it around to discover how it best fits with the unique contours on your face as well as your body. All the sides, edges, teeth, grips, and notches can be used in myriad ways, so have fun discovering and being creative.

Jade

SOOTHING • HEALING • ACTUALIZING

COLORS: Most commonly jade is a pale green. Nephrite Jade can be white, light green, dark green to almost black. Jadeite Jade can be purple, light green, dark green to almost black, lavender, yellow, or white.

ORIGIN: Jade has been in use since Neolithic times (3500–2070 BCE), when it was the crystal of choice for the Wu, the spiritual ancestors of the Taoists, in Zhejiang province in China. Jade was carved into many forms ranging from hair combs to pendants to weapons to wall carvings. Jade artifacts have been recovered from many tombs, where they were thought to escort royalty into the afterlife. Aztecs and Mayans used jade to communicate with their gods.

HEALING PROPERTIES: Jade is revered for treating the kidneys and in ancient China it was used as a remedy for kidney stones. It is also associated with the heart and is known for opening wisdom deep within. It is believed that jade balances the fluids in the body and centers the pH balance.

OFFERINGS: As a symbol of serenity and healing, jade is known for offering mental stability, soothing the nervous system, and for actualizing the most authentic self.

SKIN ENERGY: Reach for jade when you would like to remind yourself that you know yourself better than anyone and you are your greatest healer.

REGIONS: USA, Italy, Middle East, Russia, China, Myanmar

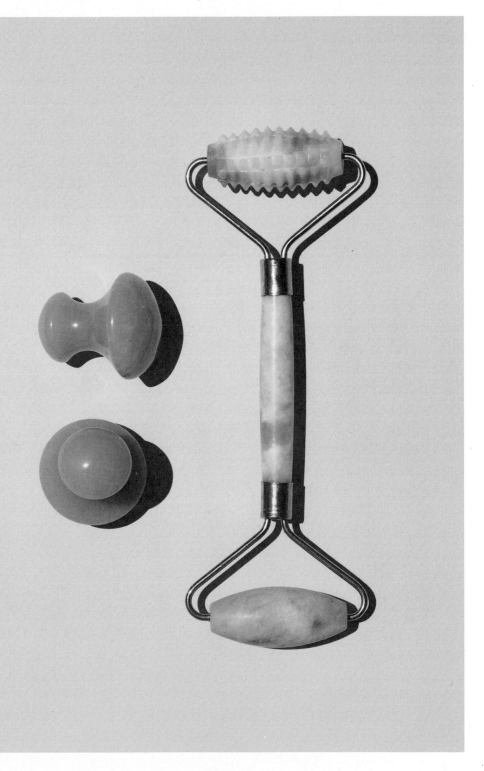

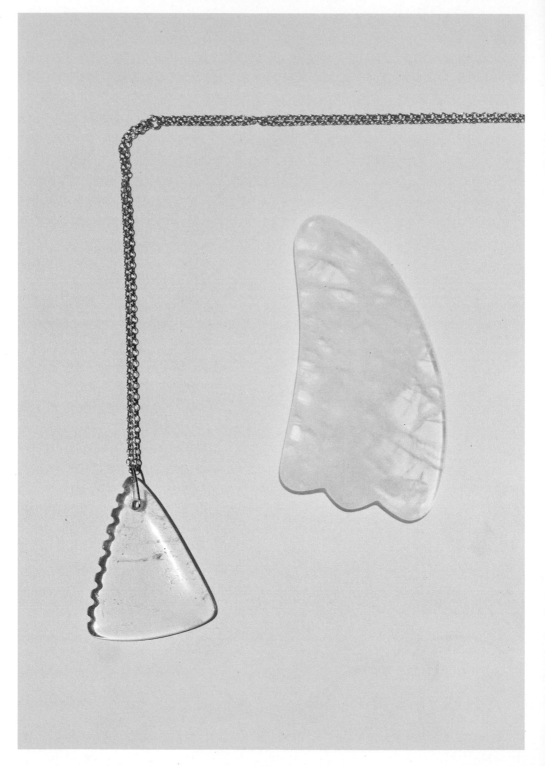

Clear Quartz

CLEANSING • ALIGNING • CLARIFYING

COLORS: Clear, milky white

ORIGIN: Both the ancient Sumerians (c. 4000 BCE) and the ancient Chinese (c. 3300 BCE) used clear quartz in their healing formulas. The Chinese character for clear quartz includes three suns, symbolizing a trinity of light. In 200 CE, the Chinese emperor was grieving the loss of his queen and an advisor surrounded the emperor with clear quartz to aid him through the heavy time.

HEALING PROPERTIES: Thought of as a cleansing gem, clear quartz is kept close to the body to aid in flushing toxins, clearing inflammation, and dispelling mental fog. Clear quartz is thought to initiate easy and clear decision-making.

OFFERINGS: The ancient Chinese believed clear quartz was the perfect jewel, symbolizing spaciousness, purity, and availability. Containing all colors of the spectrum, it aligns all levels and aspects of being at once, harmonizing the four bodies. It is believed to have the ability to return a person to the most perfect state possible: a radiant version of themselves and in perfect health.

SKIN ENERGY: Reach for clear quartz when you would like to remind yourself how to center and cleanse out any thoughts, feelings, and energies that are not yours or that you have outgrown.

REGIONS: Worldwide

Rose Quartz

UNCONDITIONALLY LOVING • WARMING • HEART-OPENING

COLORS: Pink

ORIGIN: Rose quartz beads were discovered in ancient Mesopotamia (modern-day Iraq, Kuwait, Turkey, and Syria) in 7000 BCE. Ancient Egyptians believed rose quartz could pause time and prevent aging.

HEALING PROPERTIES: Rose quartz is thought to strengthen the circulatory system by aiding in the release of impurities from the heart and pericardium.

OFFERINGS: Rose quartz is believed to assist in releasing blocked emotions and heartaches. Received as a heart-opener, it shifts grief to allow a state of loving and practiced receiving. It is thought to attract love and harmony in all relationships and future ones to come.

SKIN ENERGY: Reach for rose quartz when you would like to remind yourself to soften and apply extra loving care.

REGIONS: USA, Brazil, South Africa, Madagascar, India, Japan

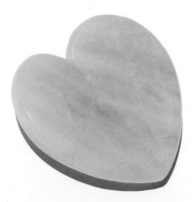

Amethyst

ALCHEMIZING • CLEARING • UPLIFTING

COLORS: Dark purple to lavender

ORIGIN: Tutankhamen's tomb, in Egypt, contained a scarab beetle bracelet carved from amethyst dating back to nearly 3000 BCE.

HEALING PROPERTIES: Often thought of as a blood cleanser, an aid to fertility, and a hormone balancer, amethyst is carried close to the body to aid all these aspects. In energy healing, amethyst is placed on the body to integrate the physical, mental, emotional, and spiritual bodies because the color purple is associated as the highest vibrational color on the spectrum.

OFFERINGS: Symbolizing the companion on a rapid spiritual journey, amethyst is known for clearing mental fog, protecting from energetic densities or heaviness, and transmuting into more authentic and evolved versions of the self.

SKIN ENERGY: Reach for amethyst when you would like to remind yourself that you have all the wisdom and answers within.

REGIONS: Canada, USA, Mexico, Brazil, Uruguay, Great Britain, East Africa, Russia, India, Sri Lanka, Siberia

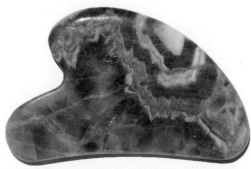

Facial Oils

Massaging oil into the skin before tracing with a gua sha tool allows the tool to slip rather than tug or pull on the skin. The gua sha tool also actively presses the serums and oils into the skin, inviting deeper layers to drink the hydrating and nourishing formulas instead of the oil evaporating or disappearing with the body's sweat.

Carrier oils

A carrier oil is a base oil or a foundational oil that comes from flowers, vegetables, or seeds that an herbalist or chemist can then blend a few more ingredients into, such as essential oils, peptides, or acids. So many clean, nontoxic facial oils are available that choosing one can feel overwhelming. Here's a breakdown of oil ingredients and options so you can discern which is best for your skin.

Tips

* If you do not eat an oil in your diet, do not put it on your skin. Our bodies absorb around 70 percent of every topical product we massage into our skin. Studies with sunscreen have discovered their ingredients (toxic and non) in the bloodstream within 20 minutes of application.
* I do not recommend massaging coconut oil into your face, neck, or chest. It is a comedogenic oil, meaning it can congest the pores, causing more buildup and potential for breakouts.

Camellia Oil: This mildly astringent, anti-inflammatory oil is high in antioxidants and omega-6 linoleic fatty acids, making it a potent skin food. It blends and absorbs into the skin easily. Camellia comes from a tea plant that is harvested to make all the caffeinated teas: green, white, oolong, and black.

Jojoba Oil: Hydrating, antibacterial, and with a mild aroma, jojoba oil mimics the body's own sebum, so it absorbs quickly and easily. Being high in iodine, jojoba is antibacterial and naturally has a very long shelf life. Jojoba is a rounded-leaf bush and the oil is extracted from its waxy seed.

SQUALENE FROM OLIVES

This is not technically a carrier oil. People with perioral dermatitis can significantly worsen the condition when treating with oils, creams, or topicals of any kind, even when they are clean and nontoxic. For some, a simple squalene oil sourced from organic olives can be relieving, nourishing, and hydrating without aggravating or spreading the inflammation further. Look for one with the single ingredient sourced from organic olives.

Olive Oil: Repairing, nourishing, and gentle, olive oil is high in antioxidants, offering rejuvenation at the cellular level and is suited to sensitive skin as it is very mild and gentle. Olives are pitted fruit from bushes and trees.

Rose Hip Oil: Rose hip oil is very gentle and usually great for sensitive skin, absorbing quickly. It softens and soothes the skin, especially mature, dry, prone-to-wrinkling skin. Refrigeration is best for this oil, once opened. Rose hips are in the rose family, growing on bushes as ripening fruit in orange to red colors.

Sea Buckthorn Oil: Anti-inflammatory, nourishing, and expediting wound healing, sea buckthorn oil is a rich nourishment for the skin, containing vitamins, minerals, antioxidants, and flavonoids. Sea buckthorn is a flowering, leafy bush that bears orange fruit resembling kumquats or orange cherry tomatoes.

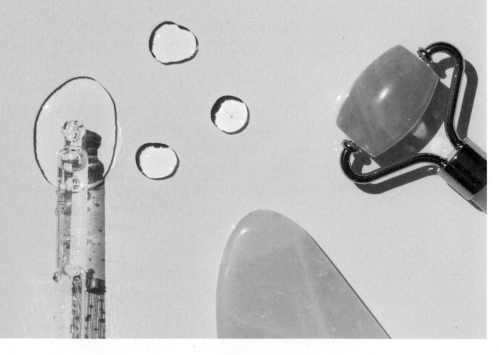

Cleaning & Cleansing Crystal Tools

It is important to work with clean tools, hands, and skin. There are two ways to clean crystal tools: physically cleaning and energetically cleansing.

Cleaning

After completing a gua sha ritual, wash your gua sha tool. There are two options for cleaning to avoid bacterial buildup:

* Wash with mild soap and water and dry with a towel. Be aware of how slippery the tool can get with soap and water and keep a firm grasp of it, as it will likely crack or shatter if dropped in a basin or on a tile floor.
* If you cannot access soap and water, wipe your tool using an alcohol wipe and then dry with a towel.

Cleansing

With repeated use, a crystal will take on a good deal of energetic information. It may absorb whatever is released emotionally during a massage and can transfer that to the body during the next session. For this reason, it is important to cleanse crystal tools and there are several ways to do this.

* Speaking to a crystal to clear it is very effective, using whatever words feel best. For example: "Clear quartz crystal, thank you for your support, you are now energetically cleansed and cleared completely."
* Another crystal can act as an energetic cleanser when placed beside a gua sha tool. Clearing and cleansing crystals include selenite, smoky quartz, and clear quartz.
* Placing a crystal tool on a the windowsill or outside beneath a full moon will cleanse it. This will also "recharge" a crystal that has given out much energy, protection, and healing.
* Smudging a crystal tool by burning sage or palo santo works to energetically clear it out. Simply light a tiny bit of sage, open a door or window, and waft the smoke all around the crystal.

DAMAGED TOOLS

Do not continue to massage with a gua sha tool that is cracked or broken. Instead, the best way to treat it is to bury it in the earth, returning it to its original home. Sometimes a crystal can burst into pieces, as if it explodes. This is truly a gift from the crystal, as it releases energy that you will not carry with you anymore.

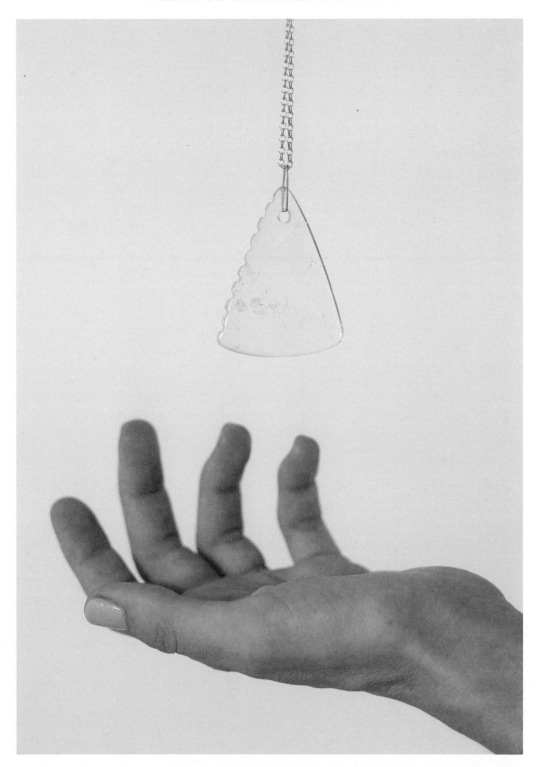

This chapter comes before we dive into the Crystal Glow Techniques (Chapter 4) because lymphatic drainage is vital to make sure that your health and wellbeing is preserved. Here we introduce very simple techniques to tend to your lymphatic system, as well as a traditional gua sha sequence (see page 46) to give us a grounding in the history of the practice.

Lymphatic Drainage & The Traditional Gua Sha Technique

CHAPTER 3

Lymphatic Drainage

A little lymph massage is always beneficial before more specific sculpting massage moves (see Chapter 4), because tending to the lymph first will help to avoid breakouts and flu/cold reactions to gua sha massage.

Everything we choose to put on our bodies is received by the blood and lymph after it travels through the skin. Sometimes this happens within seconds, or, if the molecular size of the substance is bigger, it can take 20 minutes or more. Essentially, the lymph is the immune system in watery form, carrying toxic waste from every nook and cranny of the body to be cleansed or completely released (see pages 18 and 19 for illustrations of the lymphatic system). Assisting the body with massage is the most vital and available way to support the lymphatic system, immune health, and thereby every other system of the body.

For lymphatic drainage, massaging with the hands is the most effective method. An electrical component in the fingertips offers a harmonizing charge that is lost when using tools. There are also many incredible benefits when working with tools, but I suggest working with your hands when getting to know your lymph. See page 8 if you need any help with the symbols to the left of each massage.

BENEFITS OF LYMPHATIC MASSAGE

- Strengthens the immune system

- Improves circulation

- Slims and tones

- Accelerates waste removal

- Prevents and cures swelling and bloating

- Aids digestive issues

- Redistributes glandular and node functions toward harmony

- Prevents and cures swollen tonsils

- Aids or prevents allergy reactions

- Increases radiance and glow in the skin

- Can improve senses: vision, smell, taste

Tip
* No facial oil is needed for lymphatic massage as the pressure is so faint and even the lightest graze over the skin is sensed and strongly influences the lymph.

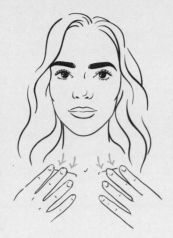

Terminus Tug

Just above your clavicles or collarbones, in the divot before the neck ascends, live the lymph nodes that cleanse all the lymph of the head, face, and neck. They are called "terminus" nodes. This massage is a good place to start a routine, activating these nodes, so they can flush before more fluid heads their way.

30 seconds

10 to 20 times

Fingertips

Ultra light to light

Stomach

Thymus, parathyroid glands, thyroid gland

With the lightest touch, and long breaths, pull at the base of your neck using your fingertips.

Give a short tug with a downward and outward motion and release.

Do not massage in circles with your fingertips because this cycles the fluids around the nodes again.

The tug notifies the nodes to function optimally in the way they were designed.

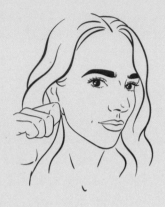

Earlobe Press

Pressing on the earlobes can stimulate a flush of the lymph for the whole head and neck. On different reflexology charts for the ear lobes, the head, sinuses, cheeks, eyes, tonsils, inner ears, mouth, tongue, jaw, and lungs are all represented. Pressing the ear lobes can also offer a centering and calming effect.

🕐 10 seconds

🔄 5 times

👆 Fingertips

🕐 Medium to deep

🖐 Triple warmer, small intestine

🧘 None

Lovingly press and pull on your earlobe, holding it between your thumb and index fingertip. You can press your earlobe between your thumb and the folded knuckle of your index finger if you prefer.

Breathe deeply and if it feels good, rock back and forth a little to assist the movement of the fluids as well as to lull your nervous system.

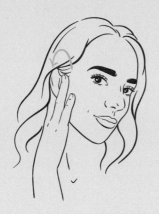

Horseshoe Press

This lymphatic drainage massage is a powerful one, so it is best not to overdo it. Flushing these lymph nodes can create a vacuum effect, pulling fluid away from the most commonly congested areas: the sinuses, the eyes, and the back of the throat. The technique can also clear fluid retained under the chin and tongue.

🕐 10 seconds

🔄 5 times

✋ Flat hands

⊙ Ultra light to light

✋ Triple warmer, small intestine, gallbladder, stomach

🧘 Thymus, parathyroid glands, thyroid gland

Breathing deeply, open your hands, extending your fingers, and make a "V" with the fingers on each hand, spreading middle away from ring fingers.

Cup the "V" under your earlobes so ring and pinky fingers are in front of your ears and middle and index fingers and thumbs are in back of your ears.

Lovingly and slowly massage in the shape of an upside down "U" or horseshoe: up, back, and down.

Avoid massaging in a full circle as this sends the fluids around and does not aid them to flush down to the terminus lymph nodes for cleansing.

If it feels good, rock back and forth a little as this gentle motion aids the movement of the fluids, softens any muscle tension to open the fluids' pathways, and offers tranquility to the nervous system.

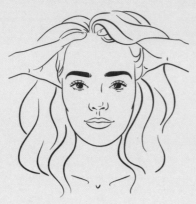

Scalp Massage

Massaging the scalp relieves tension in any of the muscle attachments at the edge of the face. It also stimulates hair growth, improves lymph flow, stimulates circulation, and clears a cloudy mind.

🕐 15 seconds

🔄 1 to 5 times

👆 Fingertips

🕐 Light to deep

✋ Governing, bladder, triple warmer, gallbladder, stomach

🧘 Pituitary gland, pineal gland

Breathing deeply, soften your jaw and move your fingertips all over your scalp.

Try massaging each fingertip in circles or spreading your fingertips wide over your scalp then drawing them back in.

Try one hand at a time, working on one side of the head and then crossing over to the other side to massage the opposite hemisphere of your brain.

You cannot go wrong, follow what feels best in the moment.

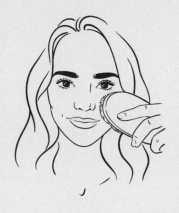

Dry Brushing

Typically, dry brushing is a technique more commonly applied to the body, using a natural bristle brush on dry skin and moving in the direction of the heart with light, swift strokes. You can dry brush your face and neck too with an extra light touch. This stimulates circulation and activates lymph movement.

🕐 15 seconds

🔄 Once

🖌 Dry brush with natural bristles

⊙ Ultra light to light

🖐 Governing, bladder, triple warmer, gallbladder, stomach, small intestine, large intestine

🧘 Lungs, stomach, large intestine, bladder, ovaries, testes, pituitary gland, pineal gland

Caution If you have had lymph nodes removed, consult with a certified lymphodema specialist or therapist for optimal DIY treatments.

With the lightest pressure, brush on your dry skin from the midline outward.

You can brush down your neck, although sometimes it feels really lovely to brush using an upward motion.

The general rule of dry brushing is to brush toward your heart.

The Traditional Gua Sha Technique

This particular sequence combines techniques from Dr. Ping Zhang, founder of Nefeli gua sha certification, from Master Jeffrey Yuen, an 88th-generation Daoist priest and Chinese medicine master, and from Five Element Chinese philosophy and acupuncture/acupressure. Each of the massage techniques in this chapter are the offspring of these traditions. Immediately we can see the benefits of these strokes to the face: from the circulation and color that enters the cheeks, to the lifting of the facial features, and the toning from releasing inflammation.

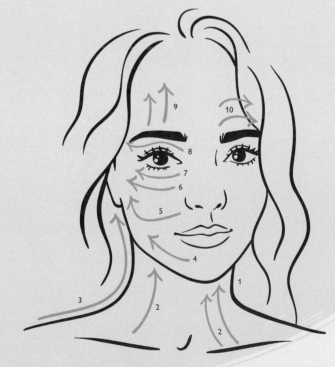

🕐 5 to 30 minutes

🔄 3 to 5 times per direction

🪶 Gua sha board
(wing/fin shape or square)

🕐 Light

🖐 All

🧘 All

Lovingly massage facial oil all over your face, neck, and the back of your neck.

Using the gua sha board "legs" or "points," hug the cervical spine at the back of the neck and trace from the base of the neck to the base of the skull. Repeat 3 times. (**1 — at the back of the neck**)

Using the flat side of the gua sha board, with as much of the tool connecting to as much skin as possible, glide upward from the collarbones—lifting the neck—to the jawline. Repeat across the entire neck, even over the Adam's apple, or larynx, with gentler pressure. (**2**)

Still using the flat side of the gua sha board, with as much of the tool connecting to the skin as possible, glide from the shoulders to the base of the skull behind the ears, massaging over the shoulder muscles. Repeat 3 times. (**3**)

Still using the flat side of the gua sha board, with as much of the tool connecting to the skin as possible, glide along your jawline from the center of your chin to your earlobes, wiggling the tool slightly at your ear to release the muscle attachments. Repeat 3 times. (**4**)

Still using the flat side of the gua sha board, with as much of the tool connecting to the skin as possible, glide beneath your cheekbone from your nostril to your ear, wiggling the tool gently in front of your ear. Repeat 3 times. (**5**)

Still using the flat side of the gua sha board, with as much of the tool connecting to the skin as possible, glide over each cheekbone from the side of your nose out toward your temple or to the top of your ear. Repeat 3 times. (**6**)

Turn the gua sha board to fit comfortably within the area beneath your eye. Lighten your pressure even more and glide from the inside corner of your eye to your hairline. Repeat 3 times. (**7**)

Turn the tool to sit comfortably over the brow bone above the upper eyelid. Glide with very light pressure, from between your brows out toward your hairline. Remaining in connection with your browbone and lift your brows up and out all the while. (**8**)

Using the flat side of the gua sha board, with as much of the tool connecting to the skin as possible, glide over your forehead from the top of your brows to your hairline, lifting upward. (**9**)

Still using the flat side of the gua sha board, glide outward over the sides of your forehead from the middle moving horizontally toward the temple and hairline on each side. (**10**)

You have the option to move straight to this chapter if you would like to start right away. Every area of the face (neck, lips, cheeks, eyes, and forehead) are addressed, so whether you want to smooth lines, relax your face, brighten your eyes, and much more, you will find a gua sha massage for you here.

Crystal Glow Techniques

CHAPTER 4

FOR THE NECK

Downward Neck Sweep

This technique sends fluids down the neck, encouraging detox by draining lymph and increasing blood circulation. Among other benefits, the technique tightens loose skin on the neck, prevents breakouts, and assists the strength of the collagen matrix or fascia. The action releases muscle tension and invites a calm spirit.

🕐 90 seconds

🔁 3 to 5 times over each area of the skin

◁ Gua sha board (wing/fin shape or square)

◢ Flat to skin and up to 20 degrees

◉ Light

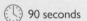 Conception vessel, triple warmer, stomach, large intestine

🧘 Thyroid gland, parathyroid glands

Caution Do not overdo this exercise, as too much can cause detox symptoms such as fatigue or nausea.

Lovingly apply facial oil all over your neck, wiping any excess onto your tool or forearms, but making sure you can still grip your tool easily without it slipping. Place your gua sha board at the top of your neck, just beneath your jaw. The tool should be completely flat to your skin.

Breathing deeply, slip your thumb underneath the bottom of the gua sha board so you can slowly glide the tool down your neck, keeping as much of the tool as possible in connection with your skin.

Apply very light pressure. The intention is to connect with the fluids, inviting the lymph to move downward, rather than to massage deeper into the muscles.

Repeat the downward stroke all the way around your neck. Use an even lighter touch when stroking downward over the larynx, the middle, and front of the neck.

Tips
- *Maintain the alignment of your spine, bringing your tool to you rather than thrusting your chin forward to greet your tool.*
- *It may help to place your fingertips above your jaw to keep the skin from pulling too much underneath the tool.*

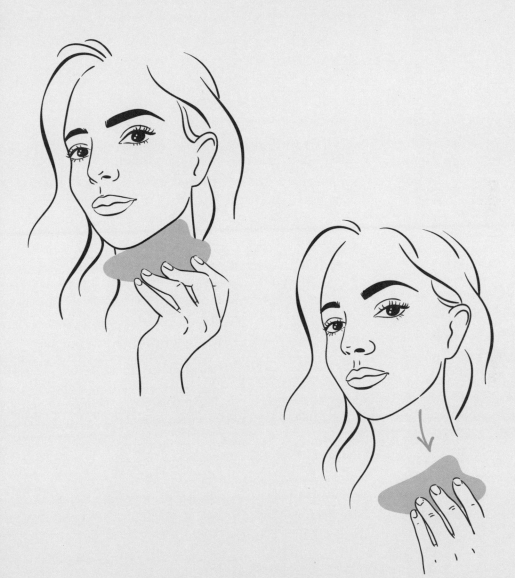

FLUID RELEASE

You may notice that you swallow several times; this is great as it means your fluids are moving. Draining the lymph in the neck allows this fluid to flush and release in the head. I've seen bags under the eyes and puffy eyelids vanish just by performing these downward strokes on the neck.

Jaw Contouring

Applying this gentle gliding move underneath the jawline assists the lymph nodes, increases blood circulation, and can shed inflammation. Benefits include a defining of the jawline, slimming of the neck, and minimizing or erasing a double chin and/or jowls. This technique also supports the voice and thyroid gland.

🕐 1 minute

🔄 3 to 10 times

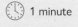 Gua sha board (wing/fin shape or square)

◁ Flat to skin

◉ Light

Conception vessel, stomach, large intestine

Lungs, thyroid gland, parathyroid glands

Lovingly massage facial oil along your jawline and underneath your earlobes. Place the gua sha tool flat underneath your chin and gently place your opposite thumb next to the tool to hold your skin taut.

Maintaining contact with the skin under your chin and jaw, glide the tool back to your earlobe. Move slowly, lovingly, while breathing deeply.

Flip the tool and offer a tender massage over those lymph nodes just below your earlobe.

Return to the Downward Neck Sweep (see page 50) to finish draining this fluid so it doesn't overwhelm the lymph nodes under the earlobes.

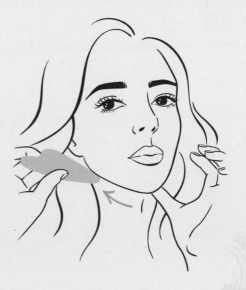

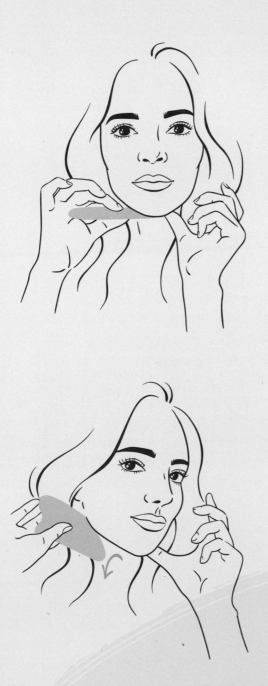

FINER LINES

This technique allows the fluid in your jowls (sagging jaw and cheeks) to drain and the lower and upper cheeks to lift up. I've seen eyelids lift and bags under the eyes diminish, or even disappear, from working this area for just a few minutes.

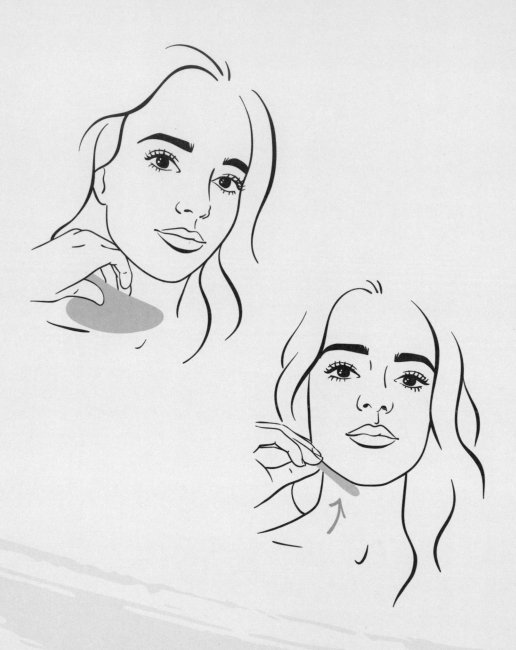

Upward Neck Sweep

Sweeping upward on the neck invites blood from the internal organs to move up into the face to nourish the cells. Other benefits include the tightening of loose skin on the neck and a strengthening of the collagen matrix. Upward sweeps also support the voice, release muscle tension, and generally uplift thoughts, mood, and energy.

🕐 90 seconds

↻ 5 times max hugging cervical spine; 3 to 5 times over the front of the neck

◠ Gua sha board (wing/fin shape or square)

◁ Flat to skin (for front of neck); 90-degree edge of "legs" (for back of neck)

◔ Medium to deep (back of neck); Light (front of neck)

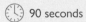 **Back of neck:** governing vessel, bladder, gallbladder, small intestine, triple warmer **Front of neck:** conception vessel, stomach, large intestine

🧘 Thyroid gland, parathyroid glands

Caution Do not overdo this exercise, as too much can cause detox symptoms such as fatigue or nausea.

Move any hair aside or put it up so that you can access the back of your neck. No facial oil is needed here. Tenderly align the edge of the "legs" of your tool on either side and at the base of your cervical spine.

Firmly glide up until you meet the base of your skull or occipital ridge. Wiggle your tool gently to release any tension. Do not massage downward; this move is only ever upward.

Repeat three to five times, moving slowly and breathing deeply all the while. If this area is very tender, lighten your pressure considerably.

Lovingly massage facial oil all over the front and sides of your neck. Place the tool completely flat on one side of your neck, just above the collarbone.

Place your thumb on the outside of the tool to steady it and slip your fingertips underneath the top of your tool and glide up your neck.

On reaching the top, turn the tool to hug underneath the jaw, maintaining contact as you follow your contours. Work slowly, breathing deeply all the while.

Comb Edge Massage

A tool with a toothed edge can treat wrinkles by breaking up the creases. This technique alleviates the patterns and tensions of held expressions, allowing the layers of your fascia to be released and rebalanced. This rapid movement stimulates the production of collagen, breaks up scar tissue, and stimulates circulation.

🕐 45 seconds

🔄 2 to 3 times

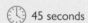 Any tool with a toothed edge

📐 90 degrees to skin

🕐 Light

 Conception vessel, stomach, large intestine

🧘 Thyroid gland, parathyroid glands

Caution If tenderness or pain occurs, stop, and take a break.

Lovingly massage facial oil all over the front and sides of your neck. Place the comb edge inside a line or wrinkle in the neck and place a few fingertips on the side of your neck holding the skin taut.

Lightly, swiftly massage back and forth horizontally into the wrinkle. Do not worry, you are not deepening the wrinkle, you are breaking up the pattern of the wrinkle. Massage back and forth for five seconds or for one deep inhale and exhale.

Rotate the tool so it is perpendicular to the wrinkle and comb up and down, all along the wrinkle, for another five seconds or the duration of another long breath.

Repeat horizontal and vertical moves two to three times, working lovingly and gently. If pain occurs, lighten your pressure or take a break and come back to it the next day.

Tips
- *Practice this technique daily or several times a week, only a little at a time. You will see results with just a one-minute daily routine.*
- *Take a "before" picture and then set a reminder in two weeks to take a "progress" photo.*

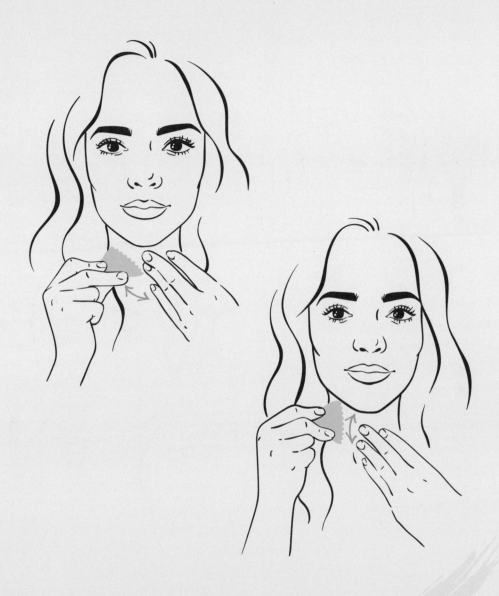

SMOOTHER SKIN

With repeated practice this technique could fill in wrinkles naturally. It can also be used on fully healed keloids (raised scars), scarring (flat scars or dimpled scars from cystic acne), and perhaps even scar tissue (scarring within the body from a surgery).

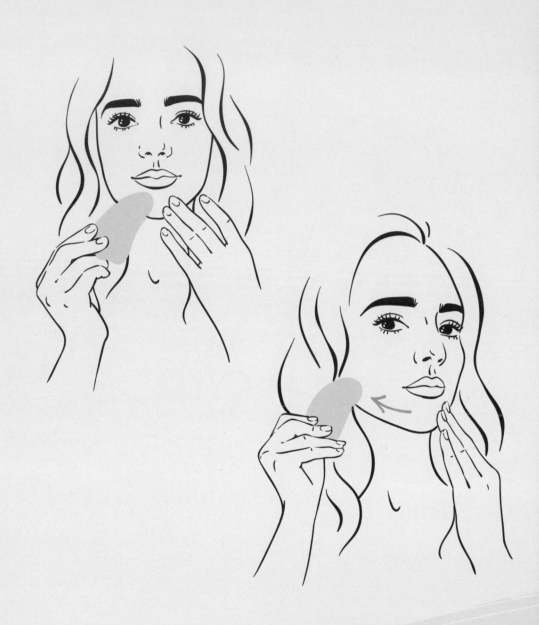

Jaw Release

Using deeper pressure to release the muscles around the jaw can prevent headaches and relieve temporomandibular joint (TMJ) disorder and its pain. Additional benefits include a defining of the jawline and a release of tension in the jaw. The technique also reduces swelling in the lower face and jaw or under the eyes.

🕐 30 to 90 seconds

↻ 3 to 10 times

◠ Gua sha board (wing/ fin shape or square)

△ Flat to skin 90 degrees (corner or point for muscle release)

◉ Medium to deep

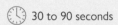 Conception vessel, stomach, large intestine

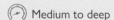 Reproductive organs, bladder, large intestine, lungs

Lovingly massage facial oil along your jawline and underneath your earlobes. Place the gua sha tool flat in the center of your chin.

Breathing deeply, glide the tool along your jawline toward your earlobe. You may like to use more pressure here to work in the muscles, inviting them to release.

Repeat as many times as you like, but no more than ten times in one sitting. Switch the tool to your other hand and glide along the opposite side of your jaw.

There is often more tension in the muscles toward the back corner of the mandible or jawbone. Use a point, edge, or wand tip to press into any tight areas or knots. If it feels good, move in tiny circles over each point.

Finish with a final sweep or two from the chin to the earlobe along each side of the jaw.

Tips

- *Try massaging one side of your jaw completely before moving to the other side. This way you can see the difference a few strokes can make.*
- *As you work, use your fingertips to hold the skin taut on one side of your chin, as you glide the tool to the earlobe on the opposite side.*
- *You may notice that the two sides of your jaw feel very different: one may have a lot more tension than the other. Work the side that needs it a little more, stopping as soon as there is tenderness or pain.*

FOR THE LIP

Lip Lines & Wrinkles

You can use a tool with a toothed edge to treat vertical wrinkles in your top lip, downward lines at the corners of your mouth, and smile lines at the sides of your mouth. Rapid combing activates the production of collagen, plumps the lips, melts the little lines above and below the lips, and stimulates circulation to give lips a rosy tint.

🕐 90 seconds

🔄 2 to 3 times

🪨 Any tool with a toothed edge

📐 90 degrees to skin

🕐 Light

🖐 Governing vessel, stomach, large intestine

🧘 Stomach, duodenum, small intestine, large intestine, kidneys, pancreas, adrenal glands

Caution If tenderness or pain occurs, stop, and take a break.

Only a drop of oil is needed for this technique. Dab some on your lips, smoothing it out beyond the lip line so your tool has slip outside the lips.

Place the comb edge inside a line or wrinkle in the upper or lower lip and use the fingertips of your other hand to hold the skin taut at the side of your mouth.

Lightly, swiftly massage up and down vertically into the wrinkle. Do not worry, you are not deepening the wrinkle, you are breaking up the pattern of the wrinkle. Massage up and down for five seconds or for one deep inhale and exhale.

Rotate the tool so it is perpendicular to the wrinkles and comb back and forth, all along the edge of the lip, for another five seconds or the duration of a long breath.

Repeat horizontal and vertical moves two to three times, working lovingly and gently. If you feel any pain, lighten your pressure or take a break and come back to it the next day.

Tips
- *Practice this technique daily or several times a week, only a little at a time. You will see results simply with a daily routine of less than a minute.*
- *Take a "before" picture and then set a reminder in two weeks to take a "progress" photo.*

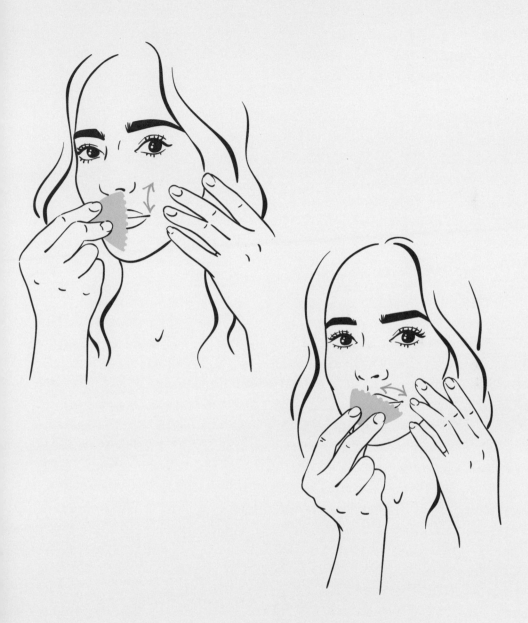

WRINKLE FILLER

With repeated practice this technique could fill in wrinkles naturally.

Lip Plumping

A lot of tension can live around your mouth. This exercise plumps the lips, lifts the corners of your mouth, and eases the muscle tension that causes drooping. The effect is to soften or erase wrinkles around lips, while inviting optimal adrenal and stomach function via the meridian lines.

60 to 90 seconds

3 times

Clean fingers

Flat to skin

Light to medium

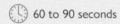 Governing vessel, conception vessel, stomach, large intestine

Stomach, large intestine

With clean hands and face, apply a very light amount of facial oil to your lips, around your mouth, and even up to your nose and the sides of your nostrils.

Slip your thumbs under your top lip all the way up where your gums meet the tissue of your top lip inside your mouth. Place your index and middle fingers just underneath your nostrils and connect with your thumbs.

Anchoring with your thumbs inside your mouth, walk your index and middle fingers out from the bottom of your nostrils and all the way through to the ends of your top lip, massaging out any tension.

Now place your index fingers inside your mouth at the corners of your smile and thumbs on the outside to connect with your index fingers. Pinch the tissue here, using more pressure if there is more tension.

This time, use the thumbs as the anchor and the inside index fingers to work the tissue on the inside of your lower lip, from the outside, toward your chin, and back again.

Tips
· *Massaging the corners of your mouth can alleviate constipation.*
· *If there are any breakouts near the nostrils, this is an indication of adrenal stress. Avoid massaging over the breakout entirely. Perhaps only work the lower lip or corners of the mouth, and only if it feels good.*

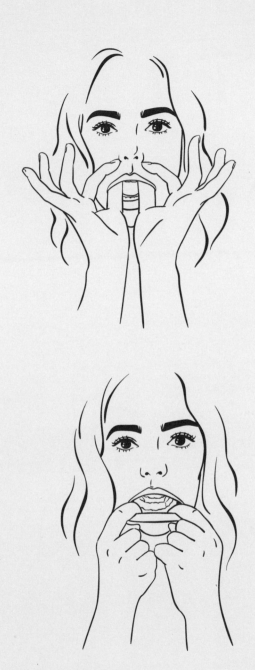

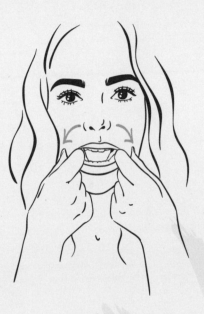

WIDE-REACHING IMPACT

Looking at the full facial chart, with this massage you are offering support to your adrenal glands, stomach, large intestine, colon, duodenum, and lungs.

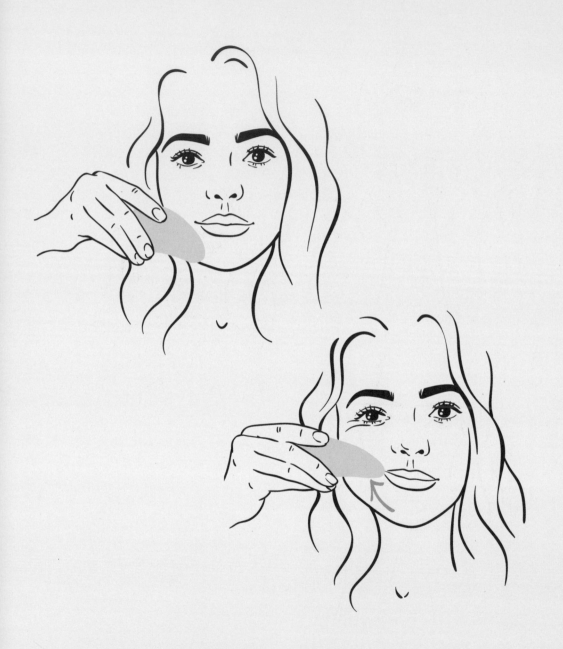

Smile Lift

The mouth is where you maintain more held expressions than other areas of the face, which can cause drooping. This technique lifts the corners of your mouth into a gentle smile, and has been shown in clinical studies to activate serotonin, dopamine, and endorphins for those who smile and see smiles.

🕐 45 seconds

🔄 3 times or more, as needed

Gua sha board (wing/fin shape or square)

△ Flat to skin

◑ Light

✋ Stomach, large intestine

Stomach, kidneys, small intestine, large intestine, adrenal glands

Lovingly apply facial oil near the corners of your mouth, on both sides.

Holding the gua sha tool flat to your skin, glide in a straight line from your jawline up to the corner of your mouth and hold in a lifted pause.

Repeat the motion three times on one side and take time to notice the difference before moving on to the other side.

Tips
- *If one side of your mouth is lower or droops more than the other, repeat this move 3 to 5 extra times on the lower side.*
- *This is half of the full "face lift" technique found on pages 76-77. If you want to extend it into the full lift, pop over and finish the technique to lift your smile, cheeks, eyelids, eyebrows, and even your forehead.*

FOR THE CHEEK

Cheekbone Sculpt

Many clients and friends have shared that their cheeks are falling, sagging, stretching down, or are very inflamed. The cheekbone sculpt technique can help with this. It clears out inflammation from lower cheeks and can eliminate jowls, while introducing contours and accentuating cheekbones.

⏱ 30 seconds

🔄 3 to 5 times

◺ Gua sha board (wing/ fin shape or square)

📐 Flat to skin

🕐 Medium to deep

✋ Stomach, large intestine, small intestine

🧘 Lungs, bronchi, kidneys, duodenum, large intestine **Left side:** Spleen, stomach **Right side:** Liver, gall bladder

Lovingly massage facial oil on your lower cheeks, jawline, and on your ears (over the tragus and earlobes).

Holding the gua sha tool flat to your skin, align the smallest part of the tool with your nostril, just underneath your cheekbone.

Relax your facial muscles, so you can scoop your cheek's tissue and guide any stagnant or excess fluids to your ear where a lot of lymph nodes live.

On reaching your ear, gently wiggle the tool on top of your tragus, to stimulate the lymph nodes to drain.

Using medium to deep pressure—whichever feels most comfortable—continue gliding from nostril to ear three to five times on each side.

Tips
· *Try massaging one side at a time to see if you can notice the difference. Do your cheekbones "pop" after a few strokes? Do your lower cheeks look slimmer?*
· *If any nausea occurs, tap or stomp your feet on the floor a few times and breathe deeply.*
· *You can also lightly massage the lymph nodes in your neck just under your earlobes to encourage the lymph to keep moving instead of accumulating.*
· *If one lower cheek is much more inflamed than the other, repeat one to three times on just that side.*

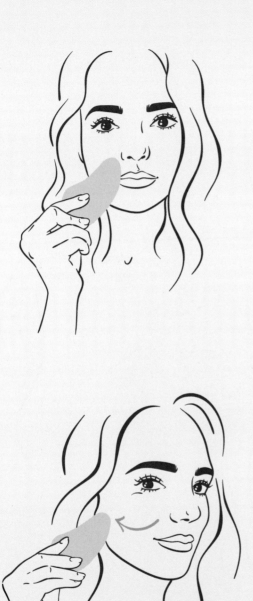

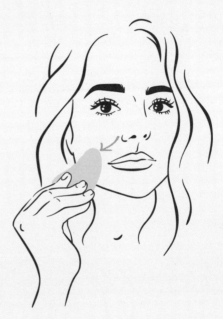

BOUNCING BACK

When we are feeling "spread thin" in our lives, our skin will stretch, and it seems to me it's an accommodation our largest organ makes for us. The move alleviates emotional burden from the skin, allowing it to "bounce back" and release its holding pattern on excess fluid so the jawline is accentuated and the lower cheeks are contoured and slimmed.

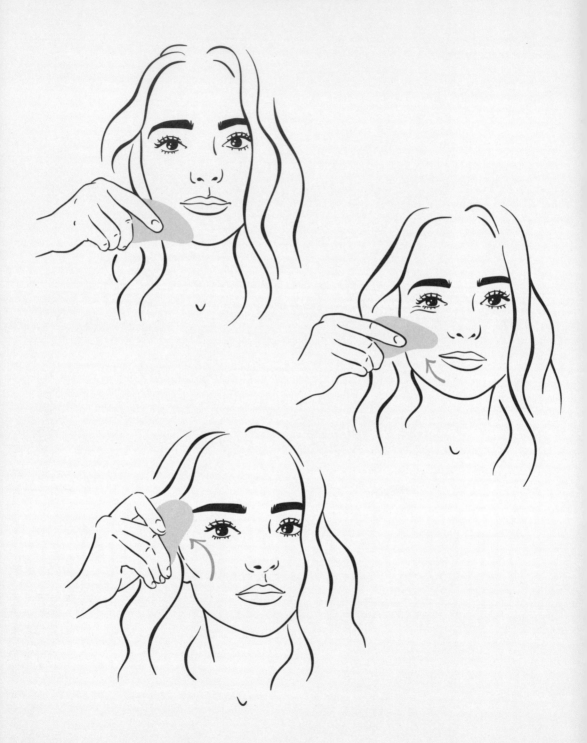

Cheek Lift

Any lifting motion on the neck and face is an instant mood elevator. The lift invites all that nutrient-rich blood from the internal organs up into the face to nourish, add rosiness to the cheeks, and stimulate the eyes. This move can feel like a face lift and is a great technique to use before an event that requires positive energy and motivation.

🕐 1.5 to 2 minutes

🔄 3 to 5 times

🪨 Gua sha board (wing/fin shape or square)

📐 Flat to skin

🕐 Light to medium

✋ Stomach, large intestine, small intestine

🧘 Lungs, bronchi, kidneys, duodenum, large intestine **Left side:** Spleen, stomach **Right side:** Liver, gall bladder

Lovingly massage facial oil over your entire cheeks, jawline, under your eyes, and on your temples.

Hold the gua sha tool flat to your skin at your jawline, your fingertips gripping the top of the tool. Start to trace upward from your jaw and over your cheekbone. Before reaching your eye, make a 90-degree turn and carry on up over your temple.

As you practice this technique, scoop up your cheek's tissue with the intention of lifting it up and out. The key is maintaining the connection and scoop of your cheek while rounding the contours of your face.

If you lose the connection—that is, if your cheek falls underneath your tool—start again at your jawline and scoop up and out. Repeat across your cheek, working your way back toward the end of your jawline and ears.

Tips
- It may feel nice to finish this technique with one or two very light sweeps under your eyes, to clear out any fluid that may have gathered there from all that movement in your cheeks. See Under-Eye Sweep, page 78.
- Breathe deeply throughout this exercise, focusing on your exhale. If images or memories arise, exhale them out of your body for clarity, greater perspective, and then full release. If a lot of grief is coming up to clear, it may feel supportive to rock from side to side or let your back release into the back of a chair or the wall.

Cheek Texturing

This technique requires a roller tool with both a textured and smooth end. The steps release tight muscles and rebalance the relationships between the layers of fascia, the muscles, and the fluids, to bring a smoother texture to the outermost layer. It can eliminate jowls, soften or eradicate tension, and aid digestion.

1 minute

Once with each roller end

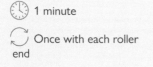 Face roller (with both a textured and smooth roller)

45 degrees, adjusting intuitively for comfort

Light

 Stomach, gallbladder, small intestine, large intestine

Lungs, bronchi, kidneys, duodenum, large intestine **Left side:** Spleen, stomach **Right side:** Liver, gall bladder

No facial oil is needed when using a roller. Place the roller's textured end on your skin. Visualizing a connection with all the layers beneath the surface, roll lightly and vigorously in any and all directions to increase blood circulation all over one cheek.

Pay attention to the areas of your body that are addressed using this technique. If there is an area of tension, roll a little extra there or apply a bit more pressure. Notice what feels good and back off if it's too much.

After a few seconds, flip your roller and place the smooth end on your cheek anywhere near the midline of your face and slowly, lightly roll from the center of your face out toward your hairline to send the lymph outward.

Experiment working slowly and lovingly, as well as vigorously, while breathing deeply when using the smooth end of the tool. Switch to your other cheek, noticing how one side feels compared to the other.

Tips
- *You can sub a gua sha board with a toothed edge for the rolling tool, but massage oil on your cheeks before you begin. Keep the pressure extra light while using the toothed edge and only make movements from the midline of your face, across your cheeks, and toward your hairline (not in any direction as with the roller).*
- *Offer yourself a moment after you complete this technique to observe any changes in the texture of your cheeks.*

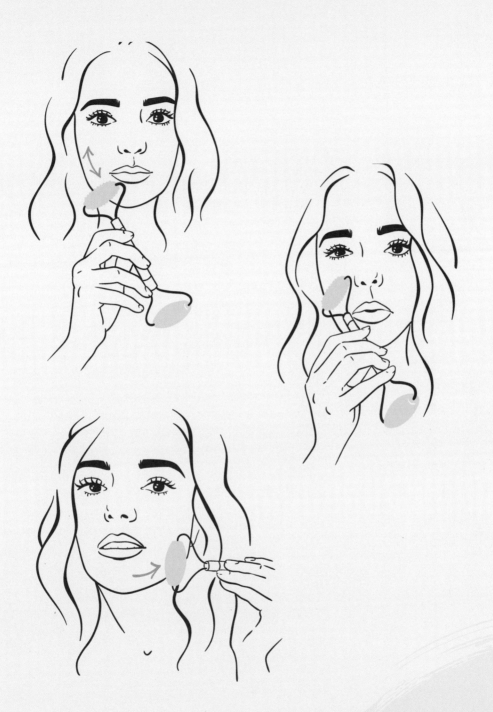

Cheek Muscle Release

Releasing the nasalis muscle can alleviate sinus pressure, seasonal allergies, and flu/cold congestion. This deeper tissue massage invites deeper and easier breaths, a widening in the corpus callosum (bridge between the brain's hemispheres), softens the muscles around the eyes, and can rid under-eye bags.

 30 seconds

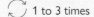 1 to 3 times

 Gua sha board (wing/fin shape) or spoon

 90 degrees

 Deep

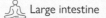 Large intestine

Large intestine

Using your fingertips, search around for the nasalis muscle, on either side of the bridge of your nose. If you trace outward from the nasal bone, it's the first muscle bump you greet before gliding over your cheekbones and orbicularis oculi muscle (the muscle that moves in a circle around your eye and extends across the top of your cheeks).

Lovingly massage a drop of facial oil over the nasalis muscle and place the edge of the gua sha board or the tip point of the spoon at 90 degrees into this tissue.

Massage outward a millimeter with deeper pressure or it may feel good to massage in a tiny circular motion with the tip point of the spoon.

Breathe deeply and back off if there is too much tenderness.

Tips
- *Follow this technique with the Cheekbone Clear on pages 74–75 for a nice way to finish and guide the lymph and blood you've just stimulated from this muscle.*
- *Notice your inhale after completing this technique. Does your breath feel wider or more available? Has your sense of smell changed?*
- *You may want to blow your nose after this technique because the muscle release may have dislodged some old gunk!*

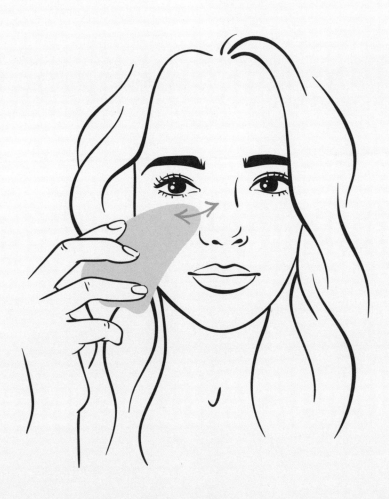

Cheekbone Clear

The upper cheeks, over the cheekbones, represent the large intestine, and the more you can clear fluid from here, the more support you give to the large intestine. This technique aids breathing, lifts emotional heaviness, and detoxes lymph stagnation in the upper cheeks and around your eyes.

🕐 30 to 45 seconds

🔄 3 to 5 times

🪨 Gua sha board (wing/fin shape)

📐 Flat to skin

🔘 Light

✋ Stomach, small intestine, gallbladder, triple warmer

🧘 Large intestine, adrenal line (only if visible), spleen, kidneys

Lovingly massage facial oil on your upper cheeks, under your eyes, and on your temples.

Place the flat side of your gua sha tool on your upper cheek next to the bridge of your nose, then glide outward with a very light touch over your temples and toward your hairline.

Repeat a few more times while breathing deeply.

Tips
- *If you have sinus pressure, try the Cheek Muscle Release on pages 72-73, and finish a smoothing stroke afterward with this Cheekbone Clear.*
- *Apply this move a few more times to one cheek if it feels tighter or more congested; it will help to release any buildup.*

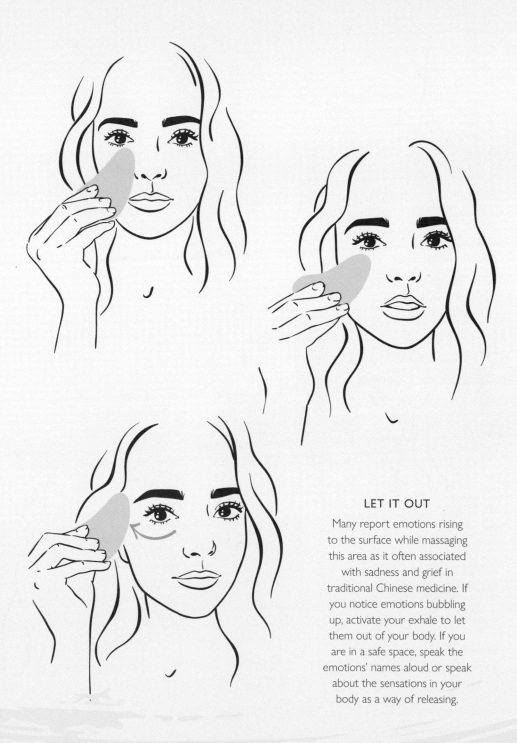

LET IT OUT

Many report emotions rising to the surface while massaging this area as it often associated with sadness and grief in traditional Chinese medicine. If you notice emotions bubbling up, activate your exhale to let them out of your body. If you are in a safe space, speak the emotions' names aloud or speak about the sensations in your body as a way of releasing.

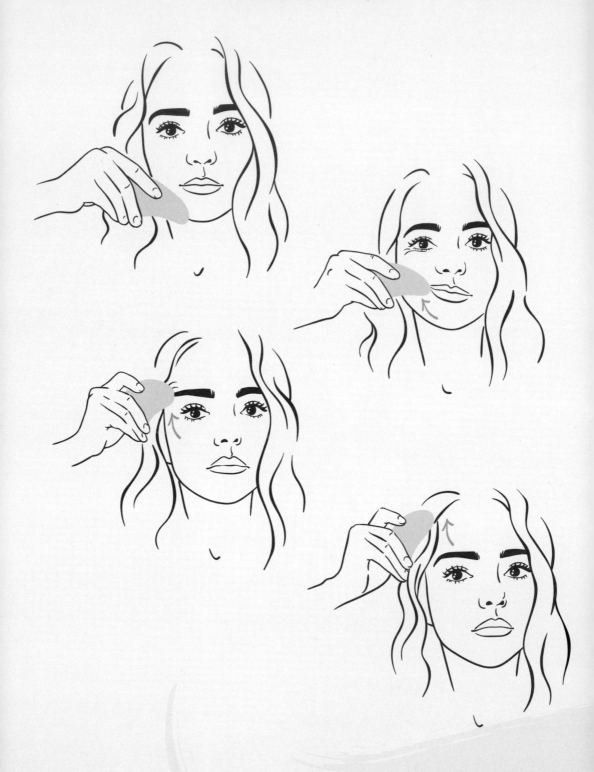

Face Lift

This single stroke can lift the entire face and expression in one move. Following the stomach meridian, with two pauses for extra lift, this technique can offer the results of five techniques in one. The action lifts the corners of your mouth, your cheeks, eyes, eyebrows, and forehead. It may also increase energy and metabolism.

🕐 20 to 60 seconds

🔄 1 to 5 times

◁ Gua sha board (wing/fin shape)

◿ Flat to skin

◉ Light to medium

 Stomach, small intestine, large intestine, gallbladder, triple warmer

🧘 Lungs, large intestine, kidneys **Left side:** Stomach, spleen **Right side:** Liver, gallbladder

Lovingly massage facial oil all over your face, including your jawline.

Place your gua sha board flat to your skin at your jawline, lining the tool up with the corner of your mouth.

Glide the tool, scooping up from your jawline to the corner of your mouth. Pause here in a lifting motion, then trace outward over the contours of your cheek to the end or arch of your brow.

Pause again in a lifting motion, then finish the lift over your temples and forehead out to your hairline.

Repeat on the other side.

Tips
- *If one side of your face is lower or droops more than the other, repeat this technique 1 to 2 times more on that lower side to invite symmetry.*
- *This technique is great for those short on time, who need a quick pick-me-up, have a photoshoot, or are about to leave for a date, for example.*

FOR THE EYE

Under-Eye Sweep

Gliding underneath the eyes supports the eyes so they are not
dragged down, or pulled up in surprise or when stress levels are high.
This incredibly gentle sweep is a lymphatic detox, a muscle support,
and a tension release all at the same time. It also aids in de-puffing
the area under the eye, all around the eye, and even the nose.

 15 to 20 seconds

3 times

Gua sha board (wing/fin
shape)

Flat to skin

Incredibly light

Stomach, gallbladder,
triple warmer

Kidneys

Caution The under-eye
skin is the most sensitive on
the face, so be tender and
gentle here. Avoid oil in your
eye, and keep the tool and
your hands and skin very
clean when working this area.
Sometimes massage in this
area can create inflammation
under the eyes if the lymph
has not been moved in a
while. If swelling occurs,
massage with ice cubes or
simply place a chilled gua sha
tool underneath the eyes to
rid the swelling.

Lovingly massage a drop of facial oil onto your under-eye
areas, avoiding your lashes and the eyes themselves. Very
little oil is needed here, as this skin tends to be the most
sensitive on our faces.

Place your tool flat on your skin, lining it up beneath the
outside corner of your eye.

With the lightest touch, and no pressure, glide along below
your eye, moving toward the inside corner. This direction
greatly benefits the orbicularis oculi muscle, because you
are moving with the grain of the muscle, which flows to the
inside corner for both upper and lower lids.

Repeat this brief stroke a maximum of three times under
each eye, because of the sensitivity of this area. If you feel
you need to repeat it, do so later in the day or the next day.

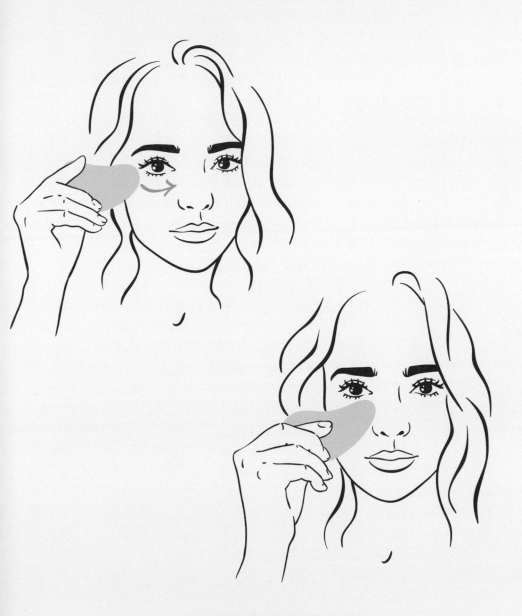

SOFTENING YOUR PERSPECTIVE

A fun exercise to try out is to try shifting your vision to allow the world to fall into your eyes. It's a gentler, fuzzier way of receiving the world and how our eyes greet what we see around us. Notice if there are any differences and how they feel.

Crow's Feet Wrinkle Eraser

You can use a tool with a toothed edge to treat horizontal wrinkles at the corners of your eyes. This technique allows the layers of tissue to refresh instead of deepening the wrinkles from repeated facial expressions. Rapid combing activates the production of collagen, filling in lines, and stimulating the circulation around your eyes.

🕐 30 seconds

🔄 2 to 3 times

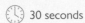 Any tool with a toothed edge

📐 90 degrees to skin

🎯 Light

✋ Stomach, gallbladder

🧘 Kidneys, gallbladder, ovaries, testes, breasts

Caution If tenderness or pain occurs, stop, and take a break.

Lovingly massage only a drop of oil to the outside corners of your eyes, where smile lines may live.

Place your thumb on your cheek below your eye and place your index finger above your eye on your forehead, then pull skin taut between your fingertips so the crow's feet area isn't wiggly.

Starting just below your eye, place the toothed edge of your tool inside a line or wrinkle and move back and forth in a horizontal motion, while working up toward a spot level with your eyebrow. Continue to massage back and forth for five seconds or for one deep inhale and exhale.

Rotate the tool so it is perpendicular to the wrinkles and comb up and down, again, for five seconds or the duration of a long breath.

Repeat these horizontal and vertical moves two to three times, working lovingly and gently. If you feel any pain, lighten your pressure or take a break and come back to it the next day.

Tip
· *Practice this technique daily or several times a week, only a little at a time. You will see results with a daily routine of less than a minute.*

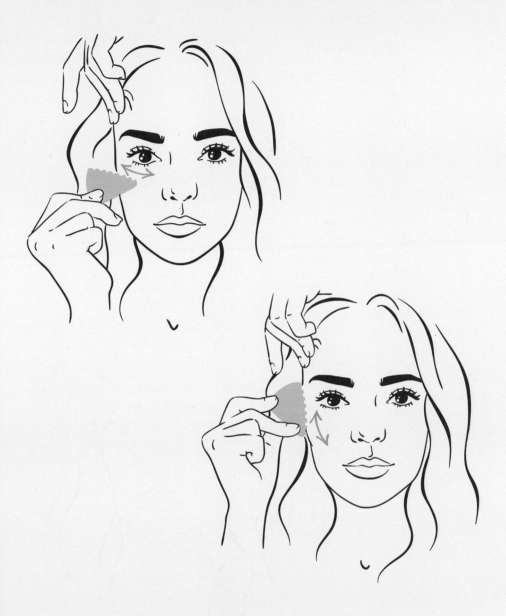

ERASING THE PAST

The section of your face that includes your eyes, temples, and bridge of your nose often represents how you lived in your 30s. The shape and depth of the crow's feet lines can reveal the stories from this decade of your life. Combing this area is a beneficial way of letting go of any experiences you've outgrown or ones you don't wish to carry on your face anymore.

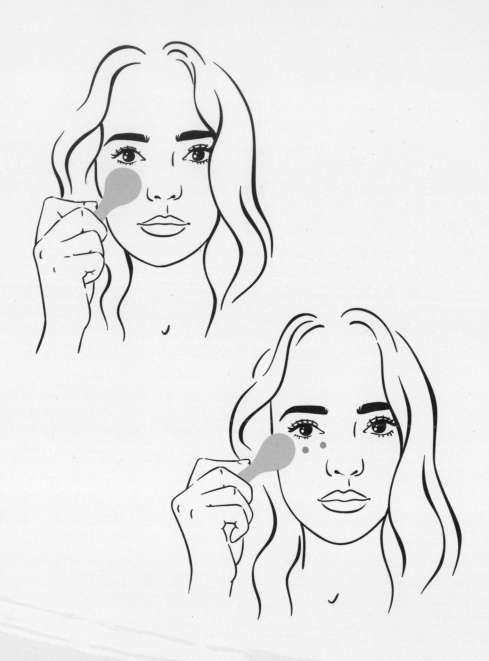

Eye Press

This is exactly as it sounds: instead of a massage or technical guide, this is a simple use of pressure to constrict the blood vessels with a chilled tool and to rush the lymph fluid out of the under-eye area that can build up during sleep. This press can eradicate under-eye bags, any puffiness around the eyes, and discoloration or redness.

45 seconds

Once

Gua sha board (wing/fin shape) or spoons

Flat to skin

Light

Stomach, gallbladder

Kidneys, gallbladder, ovaries, testes, breasts

Chill your gua sha tool in the refrigerator, or even in the freezer, overnight or for a minimum of 15 minutes. (Do not put a frozen or chilled gua sha tool under hot water, it can crack.)

Dab the chilled tool to your under-eye to acquaint this sensitive skin to the cold temperature of the tool.

When ready, place the tool flat on your skin beneath your eye.

Inhale and exhale slowly then lift the tool and place it in the next spot under-eye and continue until both under eyes have experienced the chilled tool for long inhales and exhales.

Tips
- *You may need to refrigerate the tool again mid-technique if there is a lot of heat coming off your eyes. Chilling two tools can be useful for this.*
- *You can use ice cubes made from spring water or green tea instead of a gua sha tool. The caffeine in the green tea will offer more constriction in the blood vessels and the antioxidants will nourish the skin's layers.*

Eyebrow Lift

This brow sweep brings relaxation to your whole body. Lifting and gently massaging the eyebrows is supportive to the gallbladder and fallopian tubes, and emotionally aids in shedding over-responsibility and overthinking or excessive worrying.

🕐 40 seconds

🔄 5 times

Gua sha board (wing/fin shape)

◺ Flat to skin

🧭 Light

🖐 Bladder, stomach, gallbladder, triple warmer

🧘 Liver, gallbladder, ovaries, fallopian tubes, testes, breasts

Lovingly massage a drop or two of facial oil into the brows and temples. You don't need much.

Place the gua sha tool on your brow bone toward the midline of your face.

Avoiding the eyeball completely, and maintaining connection with your brow bone, use the tool to lift your eyebrow and then glide the tool out over your temples to your hairline.

Breathe long and deeply while you work; it may feel nice to close your eyes.

Tips
• *For the full face-lift technique, see pages 76–77.*
• *You can also inch along your brow from the inside corner to outside tip, pressing and lifting up a little bit at a time.*
• *If one of your brows is lower than the other, repeat this technique 2 to 3 more times on that side.*

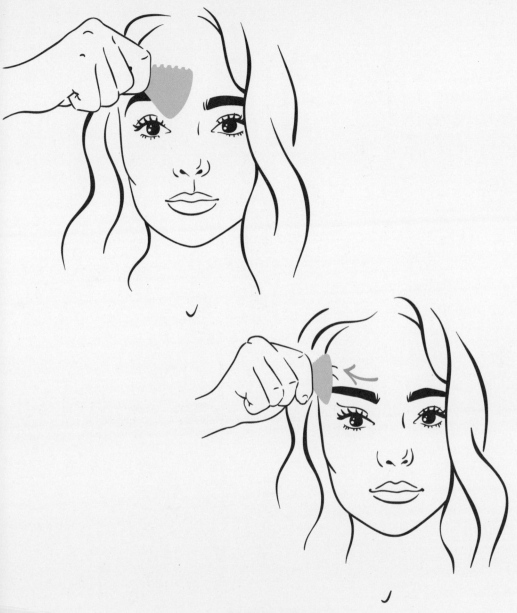

OPTIMAL HEALTH

Activate your inhales and exhales by inhaling perfect health to your
reproductive system and chest and exhaling any rage residing in your liver,
any over-responsibility or overthinking in your gallbladder, and any congestion
in your chest. Visualize your body in optimal health and harmony.

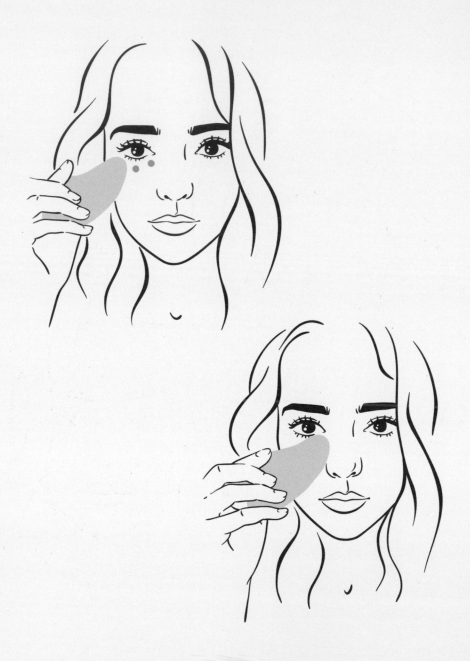

Eye Pulse

This gentle pulse stimulation aids lymph movement and drainage to alleviate puffiness around the eyes, under-eye bags, and even dark circles. This massage calms and soothes the kidneys, which is the organ that uses dark circles as a skin message for more strength and support after they've experienced too much stress and exhaustion.

Seconds

3 times

 Gua sha board (wing/fin shape) or fingertips or mushrooms

Flat to skin

Very light

Stomach, gallbladder

Kidneys, ovaries, testes, breasts

Placing your tool at the outside corner beneath your eye, gently and lightly roll the tool before lifting and placing in the next spot beneath your eye. Imagine the movement to be like the gentlest pressing of a rubber stamp.

You can also try pressing from the inside corner of your eye and working your way out to see if this feels more pleasurable. Hold the thought of remaining in the fluids instead of dragging on the muscle while you play with that direction.

Forehead Lift

Massaging the forehead is a wonderful way to begin a meditation and this technique offers an eyebrow and forehead lift, while softening lines and wrinkles. This massage may also invite clarity and aid in decision-making as you are working right over the cerebrum/frontal lobe (responsible for speech, creativity, and higher mental functions).

🕐 45 seconds

↻ Twice

◁ Gua sha board (wing/fin shape)

◿ Flat to skin

◉ Medium

 Governing, bladder, gallbladder, stomach, triple warmer

 Liver, small intestine, colon, bladder, gallbladders

Lovingly massage facial oil into your forehead and eyebrows.

Place the gua sha tool flat to your skin at one end of your forehead, over the temple, just at or above your eyebrow.

Applying medium pressure, lift up toward your hairline, continuing the lifting motion a little beyond your hairline.

Place the tool at the next spot on your forehead—on or above your eyebrow—and repeat the lifting motion.

Continue across your forehead, switching hands when you reach the center, and finishing at the opposite temple. The motion will feel rhythmic once you get going. The cross-lateral movement of massaging from left to right and then right to left (or vice versa) while switching hands, assists with brain balancing.

Repeat this process twice, switching hands and massaging in the opposite direction across your forehead.

Tip
· *Maintain the alignment of your spine, bringing your tool to you rather than thrusting your forehead forward to greet your tool. Alternatively, practice this technique lying down for total relaxation.*

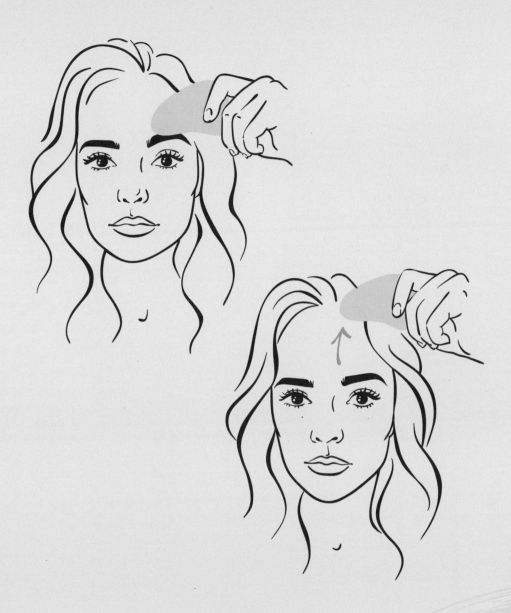

BEDTIME SOOTHER

This technique is a wonderful ritual before sleeping. I nicknamed it
"The Thought Melter" and I often feel it's like a big eraser of the day's
thoughts and journey so that your sleep may be deep and free.

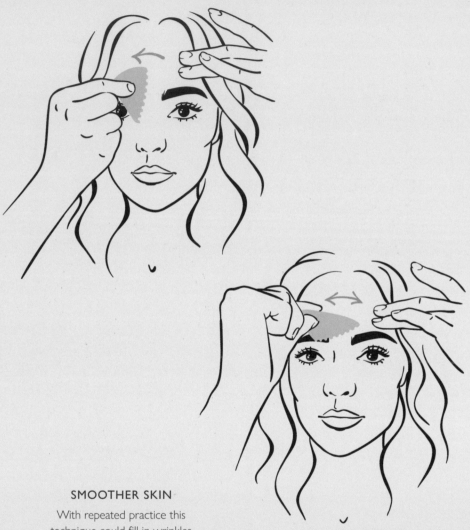

SMOOTHER SKIN

With repeated practice this technique could fill in wrinkles naturally. It can also be used on fully healed keloids (raised scars), scarring (flat scars or dimpled scars from cystic acne), and perhaps even scar tissue (scarring within the body from a surgery).

Smoothing 11s Wrinkles

A tool with a toothed edge can treat the wrinkles between the eyebrows by breaking up the creases. This technique alleviates the patterns and tensions of held expressions, allowing the layers of your fascia to be released. This rapid movement activates collagen production, breaks up scar tissue, and stimulates circulation.

🕐 40 seconds

🔄 2 to 3 times

◁ Any tool with a toothed edge

◿ 90 degrees to skin, then 45 degrees for final combing and smoothing

◉ Light

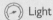 Governing, bladder

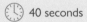 Liver, pancreas, small intestine

Caution If tenderness or pain occurs, stop, and take a break.

Lovingly massage a drop of facial oil between the eyebrows.

Place the comb edge inside a wrinkle between your eyebrows. If you don't have visible wrinkles here, furrow your brow to see where they may appear one day—this can be a preventative technique. Place a few fingertips to the side of your third eye, holding the skin taut.

Lightly, swiftly massage up and down vertically into the wrinkle. Massage up and down for five seconds or for one deep inhale and exhale.

Rotate the tool so it is perpendicular to the wrinkle and comb side to side in the space between your eyebrows. Continue for five seconds or the duration of a long breath.

Repeat horizontal and vertical moves two to three times, working lovingly and gently. Then, still using the toothed edge, angle the tool at 45 degrees and comb in the space between your brows from the midline out in either direction to inform the muscles to open outward.

Repeat this same move with the smooth side of the tool, this time flat to the skin, massaging from the midline outward in either direction. If pain occurs, lighten your pressure or take a break and come back to it the next day.

Smoothing Horizontal Forehead Lines

This technique is very similar to Smoothing 11s Wrinkles on pages 90-91. Here, however, you stretch out your movements to work on additional lines that may live across your forehead. There is more focus on the colon, especially the transverse (the part of your colon that goes across, above your belly button from right to left).

🕐 40 seconds

🔄 2 to 3 times

🪨 Any tool with a toothed edge

📐 90 degrees to skin

🕑 Light

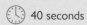 Governing, bladder

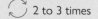 Liver, pancreas, small intestine, transverse colon

Caution If tenderness or pain occurs, stop, and take a break.

Lovingly massage facial oil onto the middle of your forehead, especially into any horizontal lines that may be there.

Insert the toothed edge of your tool into a wrinkle and place your other fingertips to the side on your forehead, pulling the skin taut.

Lightly, swiftly massage back and forth horizontally into the wrinkle. Do not worry, you are not deepening the wrinkle, you are breaking up the pattern of the wrinkle. Massage up and down for five seconds or for one deep inhale and exhale.

Rotate the tool so it is perpendicular to the wrinkle and comb lightly and swiftly up and down against the wrinkles for five seconds or one deep inhale and exhale.

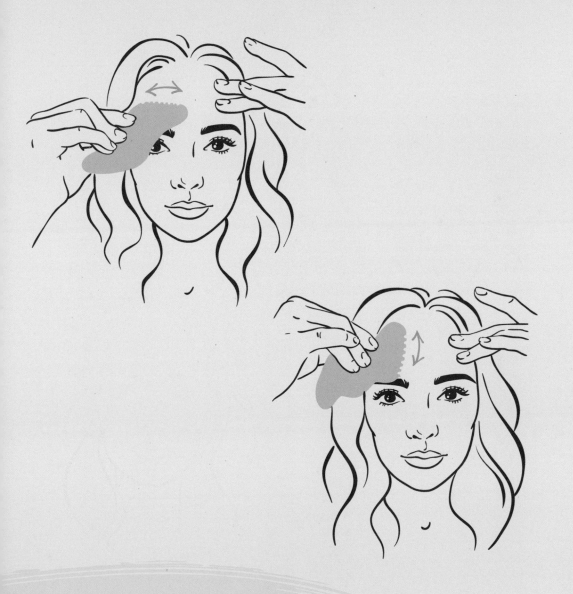

ENZYME BOOST

Taking the right digestive enzymes consistently with each meal can soften or completely erase these wrinkles. Consult with a naturopathic physician to discern if and which enzymes are best for you.

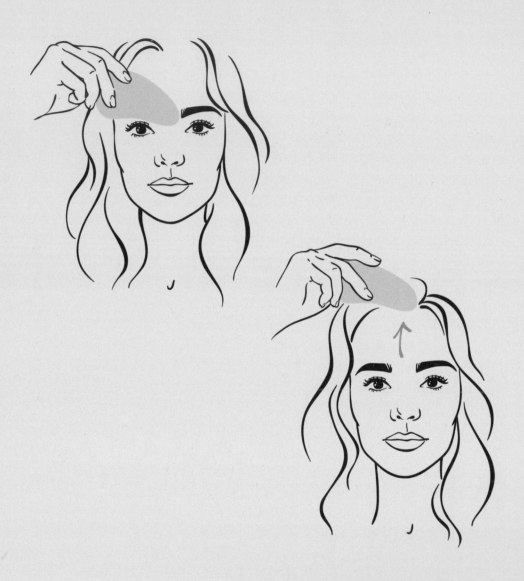

POTENTIAL FOR ENLIGHTENMENT

I have known this technique to expand the corpus callosum (the bridge between the left and right hemispheres of the brain), allowing space and new insights to flood in.

Third Eye Opener

In many cultures throughout time and around the world, using the third eye, physically and spiritually, is a practice of clear seeing or intuitive knowing. You may notice serenity washing over you and this technique can be a supportive ritual to transition into a deeper meditation practice.

🕐 1 minute

🔄 7 to 9 times

🪨 Gua sha board (wing/fin shape)

◁ Flat to skin

🕐 Very light

🖐 Governing, bladder

🧘 Pancreas, liver, small intestine, transverse colon, bladder

Lovingly, and perhaps extra slowly here, massage facial oil over your third eye and up the midline of your forehead.

Gently place your gua sha tool at the top of your nose between your brows.

With long and deep breaths, very slowly glide the tool up your forehead gently lifting off at the hairline and gently returning to the starting position between your brows.

Repeat this movement for up to 12 times.

Tips

• *Have fun exploring how slowly you can massage with this technique and how deep you can grow your breaths by the end of your movements. You could add a mantra, silently or spoken, as you work as well.*

• *Since you massaged upward on the third eye to open and expand it, it may feel nice to trace the governing meridian, which flows in the opposite direction, especially if you need to transition to something after this technique that requires focus and energy. Trace from your tailbone, up your back as best you can, following all the way up your neck, up and around the midline of your skull and down your nose to finish at your top lip.*

Comb for Muscle Release

This technique uses a toothed edge tool and is highly beneficial for soothing or even eradicating tension headaches, pain from temporomandibular joint (TMJ) disorder, and blurry vision. Once tension is released in the hairline and scalp, your forehead, eyebrows, and eyelids can lift naturally.

🕐 1.5 minutes

🔄 1 to 2 times

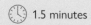 Any tool with a toothed edge

📐 5 to 90 degrees

🕐 Light to deep

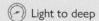 Governing, bladder, gallbladder, stomach, triple warmer

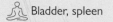 Bladder, spleen

Place the toothed edge of your tool at a 45-degree angle over one of your temples.

Applying lighter pressure over your temple, comb the skin, passing the hairline and then wiggle the tool gently into your scalp to release the muscle attachments and any buildup of tension that may be there.

Move one spot above your temple and comb again, perhaps applying more pressure now that you are off your temple. Continue past your hairline and gently wiggle the tool into your scalp in a way that feels good.

Continue across your whole forehead/hairline and, if you so choose, repeat all the way back, switching hands if that is more comfortable.

Tips
· *If you notice any tension in your jaw or neck as you work, try this technique lying down to release all those muscles.*
· *Maintain the alignment of your spine if you choose to sit or stand, bringing your tool to you rather than thrusting your forehead forward to greet your tool.*

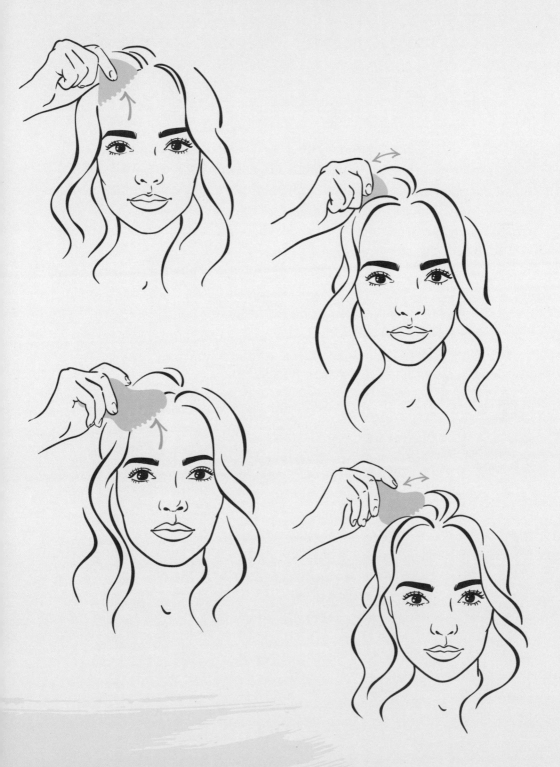

Temple Massage

Highly relaxing and deeply repatterning, working these soft points at the sides of your forehead can act like a reset button. Temporal massage or tapping is an ancient practice hailing from China, and has been used throughout time and all over in different ways for pain relief and for dissolving habits and addictions.

🕐 30 seconds

🔄 7 to 9 times

🍄 Mushrooms, spoons, or fingertips

◁ Flat to skin

◉ Very light

✋ Triple warmer, gallbladder

🧘 Spleen, kidneys, gallbladder

Caution If you start to feel dizzy or nauseous, stop and take a break.

Facial oil isn't needed here, but can feel nice for added slip between the tool and your skin.

Very gently place your tool or fingertips on both your temples at the same time and circle backward, slowly, while breathing deeply.

Continue for 30 seconds, or for as long as it feels good.

Tips

- *You can trace using a figure-eight or infinity sign over your temples. This is an additional healing technique called the "Celtic weave" or "pattern of the caduceus" (the traditional medicine symbol or the serpents weaving on Hermes' staff). This weaving or figure-eight motion has the ability to reset, restore, and heal all energy systems inside and outside your body.*
- *To break free of a habit: while you massage your temples, repeat "I am free of any and all attachments to being liked" or "I am already the person I wish to be." Keep the statements positive and in the present tense.*

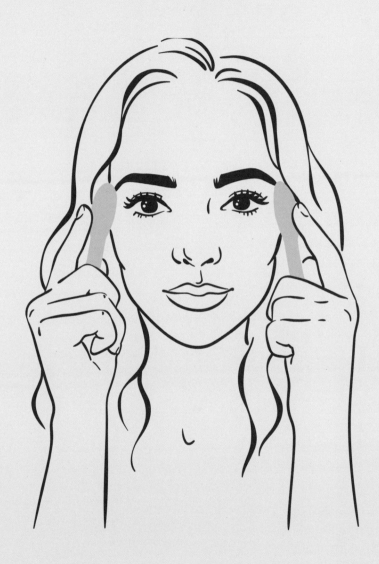

In this chapter you will find an introduction to acupressure points, which you can utilize in conjunction with gua sha massage to calm the mind, benefit the facial muscles, and harmonize the skin.

Acupressure Points to Glow Inside & Out

CHAPTER 5

Coming Back to Center: a Visualization Practice

In this chapter is an introduction to acupressure and a selection of techniques for working with your acupressure points, which can be used in conjunction with the other massage practices in this book.

Before we learn more about acupressure, it is vital to remember the concept of the "four bodies" in TCM which is the interconnectivity of our physical, emotional, mental, and spiritual selves (see page 15 for more information). For this reason, "Coming Back to Center" is a useful visualization for whenever you need it, so that you can remain true to yourself, avoid extremes as much as possible, and so that your self-care practice offers you a mind-body-spirit harmonization, in addition to all the wonderful aesthetic benefits.

In my experience, if I have thoughts regarding future worries or if I am regretting something in the past, it means I have allowed my energies to float far away from where I truly am presently. Letting myself wander into the future or past for too long spreads me too thin and is the opposite of being centered. "Coming Back to Center" means pulling my energy into the midline of my body, so that all of my strength is available and I am emotionally even-keeled. I am awake to each moment, choosing my responses wisely rather than reacting to every little thing.

YIN AND YANG AND THEIR CHARACTERISTICS

The beauty of yin and yang is that they are opposites and at the same time complementary, each holding a part of the other. This concept and symbol is an invitation to hold both and return to harmony again and again. I use the word harmony instead of balance because often I think we get caught up in the attachment that balance means equal or 50/50. Yet we are complex beings and we show up in many roles, sometimes in a single day—so instead of a balancing act, where all the cups need to be full, how about inviting harmony? Sometimes a cup may be empty because our attention cannot be everywhere at once with equal presence, and this is ok! I believe we can hold all these roles or cups and allow our attention to be where we intend, then also allow for our attention to be pulled where it is needed, even if that goes against how we had planned. I feel this allows us to be flexible rather than breaking under the pressure within us. I find moms are experts at this, growing into their own expression of harmony more and more each day (even if it's mostly because the pressures of the role demand it be so).

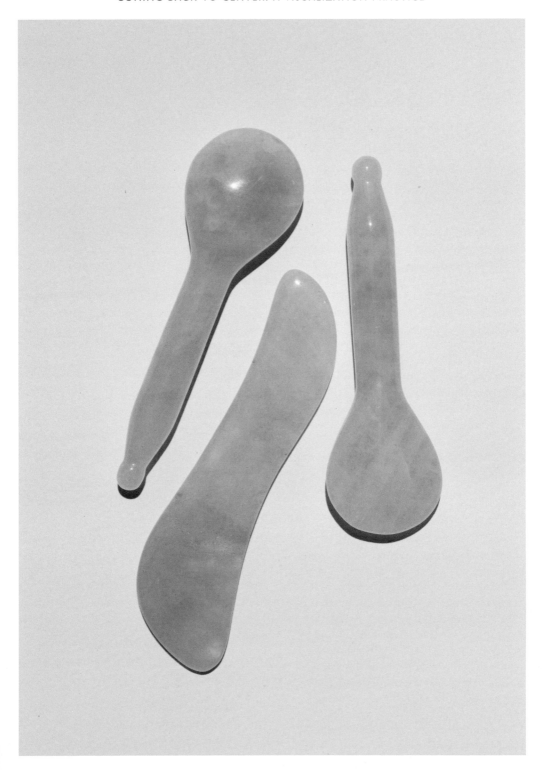

Working with Your Acupressure Points

Acupressure is an ancient practice inviting harmony and wellbeing within and all around the body. It hails from China, where records as early as 2000 BCE exist. Acupressure points live along the energy meridian paths and are conduits for electrical signals with the abilities to open up blockages in the energy meridians, unblock "qi" or "chi," the Chinese concept of energy or life force, release muscle tension, invite blood flow, and activate the points' self-curing properties. Whatever your issue, there is likely to be a "button" for it so you can address it quickly and easily.

The best tool to use when working with acupressure points is a gua sha spoon; use just the tip, which is rounded and has a small surface area. Avoid using anything too sharp or so large that the point is lost within the surrounding area. Fingertips are also ideal because they are electric and the skin-to-skin contact is healing.

The locations of the points vary because we are all different. Finding your electrical hotspots is an exercise in intuition and body listening—you truly will know it when you feel it; for some, landing on a point feels like a buzz, almost like a lightbulb switching on. Feel for a softer area, almost like an indent, and see if you notice a little activation, maybe the area is tender or perhaps it feels as if there is movement underneath the spot. Play around with a given area, pressing at different intensities to find your point.

The length of time for holding each point is up to you. In traditional practice, points can have an effect when pressing for anywhere between 5 seconds and 15 minutes. Each point has different needs and requires varying depths of pressure, so use your initial practice to discover what each point needs at the time you visit with it. If you are able, carve out some time to be with yourself without rushing so you can really listen to your body at a deeper level than perhaps ever before. For the exercises that follow, around 90 seconds is perfect with each point.

CAUTION

While trying to conceive and during pregnancy, avoid these points:

- The inner ankle point named Joyful Sleep, K 6, would be best to avoid as it can act like an "eject" point and has been known to start labor.

- The center of the diaphragm, or where the ribs fan out, named Center of Power, CV 12, ought to be avoided during pregnancy as any pressure around the abdomen is best avoided, unless during an exam by a midwife or gynecologist.

- If you are exploring other pressure points beyond the few in this book, the following are also important points to avoid during pregnancy or when trying to conceive: SP 6, LI 4, BL 60, BL 67, GB 21, LU 7, and points in the lower abdomen (e.g. CV 3–CV 7) and sacral region (e.g. BL 27–34).

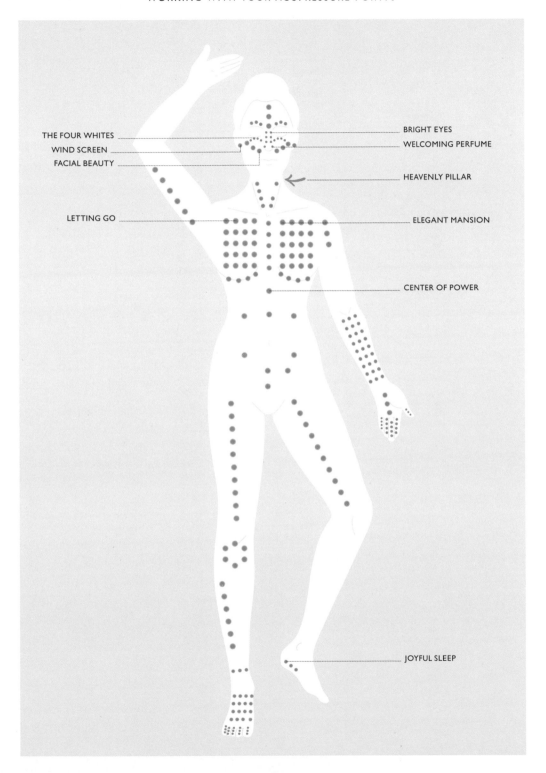

THE FOUR WHITES

WIND SCREEN

FACIAL BEAUTY

LETTING GO

BRIGHT EYES

WELCOMING PERFUME

HEAVENLY PILLAR

ELEGANT MANSION

CENTER OF POWER

JOYFUL SLEEP

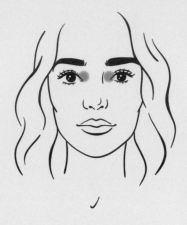

Bright Eyes

Applying the lightest pressure to these points in the corners of your eyes may alleviate, or even eradicate, eye pain and can improve vision. It can also relieve severe nosebleeds. If pressure is applied with crossed wrists—so using opposite fingertips—this point may also offer brain-balancing benefits.

Name/Association

Bl 1 = Bladder/Bright Eyes

◉ Inner eye corner, just above tear duct

◯ 2 spoons

🖐 Bladder

🧘 Ovaries, testes, pancreas, gallbladder (both sides for these points), adrenal glands

Before pressing with the tips of the spoons, find each point using a fingertip first, because the tissue is very sensitive around the eyes. Locate the hollow, or soft point, in the inner corner of each eye, just above the tear duct. You may even feel an energy shift once you land in the points.

Breathing long and deeply, gently apply a tip of a spoon into each Bright Eyes point. You can use your fingertips, if you prefer. Play with your breathing here.

Explore pressing the Bright Eyes points with your eyes closed and then with your eyes open. Try lying down as well as sitting up.

Notice what feels best in the moment, which may be very different each time you return to these points. Greet yourself as you are and where you are.

Center of Power

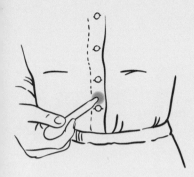

This point in the abdomen, if pressed when the stomach is not full of food, can be very calming to the whole body and all systems within. Loving pressure on the CV 12 point can relieve frustration, emotional stress, and headaches. It can harmonize the stomach and calm indigestion.

Name/Association
CV 12 = Center of Power

⊙ Middle of diaphragm where ribs fan out

 Spoon

 Conception vessel

🧘 Stomach

Caution
Avoid this point entirely if you are pregnant or if you are unwell or have a serious illness.

Do not exceed 2 minutes when holding this point.

Find the center of your diaphragm by tracing down the sternum, the bone that connects the rib cage, to where it ends, and it becomes fleshy and soft. This area should not feel tender, so perhaps move a couple finger widths lower if there is a sharp or tender pain when you press.

Using the tip of the spoon, or your fingertip, apply a medium amount of pressure and breathe deeply.

Try this in both a seated position and lying down, to see what feels best for you.

Notice which muscles soften right away, and which ones tense up. Notice if there is any release at the top of your neck where the occipital bone, the ridge at the back of your skull, meets your spine. Notice if your shoulders drop away from your ears.

Encourage your body to release by growing and expanding your breaths.

Tip
• *This acupressure point is best pressed on a nearly empty stomach.*

Facial Beauty

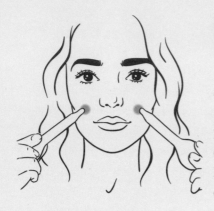

Applying pressure to these two points on the face can remedy acne and facial blemishes. Pressing these points improves facial complexion, activates blood circulation, and lifts sagging cheeks. It can also relieve head congestion, a stuffy nose, and burning eyes. It opens up the ears and can clear the sinuses and face.

Name/Association

St 3 = Stomach/Facial Beauty

◉ Under cheekbones, lining up with eye pupils

◠ 2 spoons

Large intestine

Lungs, intestines, liver (right side), stomach (left side), adrenal glands

Using the tips of the spoons, or your fingertip, locate St 3 by tracing outward from your nostrils to a point directly beneath the pupil of each eye. Apply pressure to both sides at the same time.

The points are underneath your cheekbones on either side of your face. See if you can hook your thumbs up underneath, pressing up into the bones and letting the weight of your head fall onto your thumbs.

Notice what emotions release or bubble up to the surface so that they can clear.

LETTING GO OF SADNESS

Working in the lung area of the facial map, often a lot of grief and sadness can find their exit through this point.

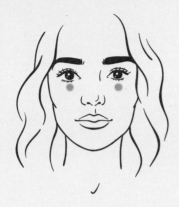

The Four Whites

These points refer to the whites of the eyes, and administering loving pressure on these points over the cheekbones can alleviate acne, facial blemishes, and burning eyes. It can also clear out the sinuses and rid the face of excess fluids and inflammation, offering a more relaxed expression and demeanor.

Name/Association

St 2 = Stomach/The Four Whites

 Over cheekbones, outward from bridge of nose

2 spoons

Stomach

Liver (right side)

Use your fingertip to locate the correct points. Trace down either side of your nose's bridge until you slide into a softer muscle over your cheek before you feel your cheekbone. Each point should align with the pupil of an eye.

Use the tips of the spoons to press into the St 2 acupressure points, on both sides of the face at the same time. This is the top of your stomach meridian. Pressure here is light, as this can be a very delicate area on the skin and is often tender in many people.

Tip

• *Use these points to clear out recent stressors from the nervous system as well as allow emotions of disgust to come up to clear. The points are powerful at releasing held memories and challenges around digesting uncomfortable events.*

FOUR CORNERS

The four corners around the mouth are also an area of consideration for the Four Whites, as skin messages showing up on the lips or corners of the mouth can reveal more about the health of the stomach.

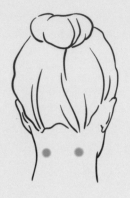

Heavenly Pillar

Situated at the top of the pillaring spine, these points carry a lot and so tending to them can mitigate and release much in the realms of anxiety, stress, burnout, overexertion, and insomnia. Pressing into these points activates the sensory organs, heightening hearing, taste, smell, sight, and touch.

Name/Association
Bl 10 = Bladder/Heavenly Pillar

⊙ Back of the neck, a few finger widths below the ridge of the skull (occipital ridge), on either side of the spine

🥄 2 spoons, although fingertips might be easier

 Bladder

 Bladder

Working these points might be easier or more pleasurable using fingertips instead of the tips of the spoons. Flip your hand upside down and place your thumb and index fingers on the back of your neck, hugging your cervical spine.

Find the points by tracing down from the occipital ridge, the base of the skull, by just a few finger widths.

If there is a lot of tension in your neck, use both hands and make circles into the points with index and middle fingers. This will melt some of the tension away, allowing for easier access to the point.

Tip
• *Working these points has the ability to relax your whole body.*

IMMUNITY BOOST

Tending to these points often can aid immune function, since there are many lymph nodes next to this area and all around your ears. Keeping these nodes accessible for the lymph is important and melting tension away is beneficial for a clear mind and flexible attitude.

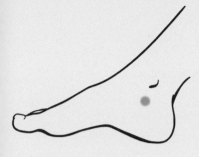

Joyful Sleep

Applying pressure to these ankle points may rid insomnia, reproductive problems, ankle pain/swelling/hypertension. These points open energy flow, clear the spirit, and calm the body. Perhaps tend to these points in bed right before you are about to sleep. Press into your Joyful Sleep points and breathe deeply.

Name/Association

K 6 = Kidneys/Joyful Sleep

◉ Below each ankle on the inside leg

◯ 2 spoons

Kidneys, spleen

Kidneys, spleen

The most comfortable position for this technique is sitting in butterfly pose, with the soles of your feet pressed together and knees splayed out. This avoids you doubling over your body to reach these points, scrunching your lungs.

Locate each ankle bone on the inside leg and slide your fingers or the tip of a spoon just below each bone, landing in the soft indentation. Press on both ankles at the same time and hold for as long as you feel is needed, or until you feel a shift within the point or in your overall being.

EMOTIONAL RELEASE

Because kidneys tend to hold the emotion of fear and the spleen tends to hold the emotions of worry or overthinking, working these points can soothe both organs and their respective emotions to allow for deeper sleep and to soften the pituitary gland so hormones are not instructed to release unnecessarily.

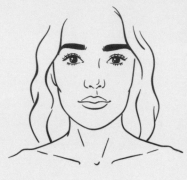

Letting Go

As the name of this technique suggests, these points allow us to release our attachments to the past and make it easier to move forward. These points clear layers of grief while strengthening our ability to take up more space by allowing our voices to be heard.

Name/Association
Lu 1 = Lungs/Letting Go

⊙ Soft chest tissue near armpits, just below collarbone

◠ 2 spoons or fingertips

🖐 Pericardium, spleen

🧘 Pericardium, spleen

About three finger widths below your collarbone, on each side of your body, the Middle Assembly points live in the soft tissue close to your armpits and above your breasts. Locate the points and press with the amount of pressure that feels good in this moment. Breathe deeply and notice if there are any sensations of "feeling lighter."

The pericardium meridian runs right underneath these points. Try working in circles to massage into the spleen meridian as well, or even into the stomach meridian if your circles are really large. Breathe deeply, and you should feel your hands rise and fall with each expansion and contraction of your lungs.

Cross your hands to press points with opposite fingers (for example, right fingertip on left chest), and you can offer your body some brain balancing, too.

EMOTIONAL OUTLET

On an emotional level, these points provide another exit point for grief and the multitude of emotions that may fall under the umbrella of grief. Often the emotion of anger is also stored in the armpit area, as we pull back our arm to throw a punch. Notice if these points stir up anger as you work, and use your exhalation to let this out of your body instead of keeping it stored in your tissues.

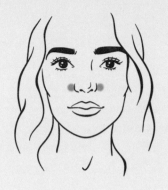

Welcoming Perfume

Pressing and spreading the nostrils open using these points on either side of the nose can eradicate stuffiness, sinus pain, and facial swelling. It can even alleviate facial paralysis.

Name/Association
LI 20 = Large Intestine/
Welcoming Perfume

Either side of the nostrils

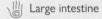 2 spoons or fingertips

Large intestine

Large intestine

Press a tip of a spoon just outside each nostril at the same time and lift outward, as if opening the nostrils to allow in more air.

Holding this opening position, breathe deeply through the nose and out through the nose.

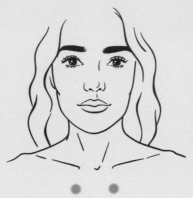

Thymus Press

These powerful reset points in the thymus can pull you out of a triggering moment. Referred to as the Shu Mansion points, they have the ability to restart the energy meridians, so that they all flow in the forward direction instead of running backward.

Name/Association

K 27 = Kidneys/Elegant Mansion

⊙ Over thymus, either side of the sternum, just below where the collarbones come together

⟋ Tips of spoons or fingertips

✋ Kidneys

🧘 Kidneys

Locate the soft indent on either side of your sternum, the bone that connects the rib cage in the center, and just below the collarbones where they come together in the middle.

If you are in a triggering moment, hold these points for a minimum of 90 seconds and remind your body to breathe as deeply as you are able.

Tip

· *These points offer a wonderful way to move through anxiety. Try this exercise as a new response to a usually stressful situation.*

A FEELING OF SAFETY

You can use just one hand on both K 27 points while using the other hand to press into the points on your forehead that protrude (about one inch above the middle of each eyebrow). This keeps the blood in your forebrain instead of it moving into your legs for flight, your arms/hands for fight, or to your center cavity for freeze.

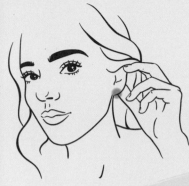

Wind Screen

This single point on each ear stimulates the lymph to flush the entire head, face, and neck so that it can alleviate acne, jaw problems, sore throats, and ear pain. These points are effective relaxants for all the facial muscles and nerves.

Name/Association
TW 17 = Triple Warmer/ Wind Screen

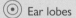 Ear lobes

Fingertips

Triple warmer

Kidneys

Press with your thumb and index finger on the front and back of each ear lobe.

To assist with detoxing the head, face, and neck's lymph, use your thumb to rub the back of each ear lobe while cupping the front with the knuckle of the curled index finger.

To alleviate tension that collects all around the ear, tug upward and outward and downward on each ear. It can feel incredibly good. Play with what you like the best.

Tip
• *This single point can be a great tool to support your immune system on a regular basis.*

We've explored each gua sha technique individually and how they interact with the organ-emotion components, so now we get to put them all together for some calming and soothing sequences that assist in creating a serene spirit and a deep night's sleep.

Cool Down Routines

CHAPTER 6

Downward Sweeps from Forehead to Neck

This relaxation sweep doubles as a lymphatic detox. It is a beneficial move to finish any sequence, as it calms the nervous system and prevents breakouts, especially if the neck has already been massaged and drained. It can also feel as if you are wiping the day from your face, setting you up for a freeing deep sleep.

Lovingly massage a few drops of facial oil onto your neck. You may also choose to use facial oil on your forehead and near your ears, but you could skip this if you do not want to grease your hair up from the oil.

Place the gua sha tool at your hairline's center and lightly sweep down toward your temple, continuing to glide down in front of your ear, and down to the base of your neck.

For the second sweep, repeat the same motion, except sweep behind your ear before sweeping down your neck.

This sequence assists all those lymph nodes around the ear and in the neck to flush out. Use light pressure and invite your breathing to deepen.

Notice the difference between the two sides of your face before moving from one side to the other.

Repeat no more than 5 times.

Tips
- *Lovingly press on Center of Power CV 12 (see page 105) to complement these downward sweeps as well as release emotional stress and indigestion.*
- *This point harmonizes the stomach and the center of your being.*

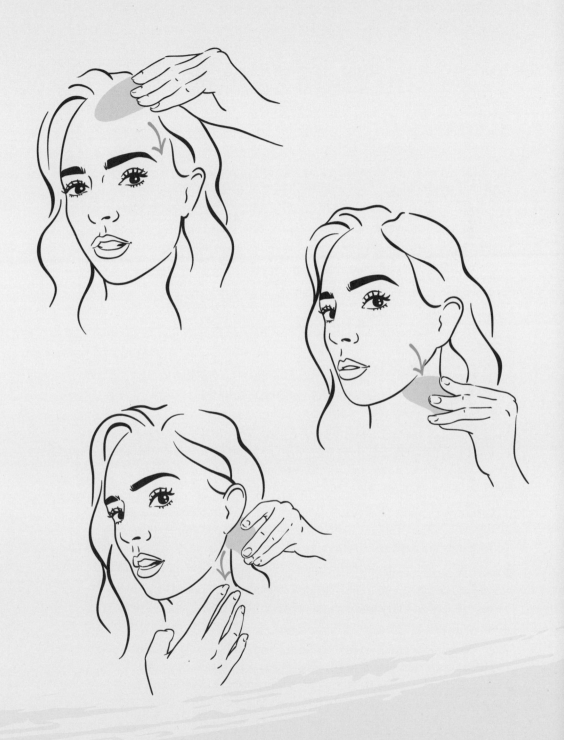

Evening Relaxation Routine

This sequence follows the reverse order to the traditional gua sha technique (see page 46)—think of it like an inversion in yoga. Moving from the top down signals to the body that it is wind-down time and you may notice your eyelids even begin to move downward and become heavy, ready for sleep.

Lovingly massage facial oil onto your forehead, cheeks, jawline, and neck.

Place the gua sha tool at the top of your forehead and, keeping the tool flat to your skin, lightly sweep from your centerline outward toward your hairline. (1)

Place the gua sha tool underneath an eyebrow toward your midline, and with a lifting motion gently glide up and out toward your hairline. Try to stay on your brow bone and do not let the tool dip into your eyelid or poke your eye. This one takes some practice. (2)

Place the gua sha tool below your eye at the inside corner of your eye. Using the lightest pressure, sweep underneath your eye and up over your temple to your hairline. (3)

Place the gua sha tool a little below where you just worked, over your cheekbone and right next to the bridge of your nose. Glide over your cheekbone using a little more pressure, yet still very light and gentle, and remain on your cheekbone all the way to your hairline. (4)

Place the gua sha tool next to your nostril and, still keeping the tool flat to the skin, trace underneath your cheekbone, massaging your lower cheek. This area can take a little more pressure. As you reach your ear, give a little wiggle with the tip of the gua sha tool. This wiggle aids the release of lymph from this area, where it may have become stuck, and supports its downward journey to the lymph nodes for cleansing. At the same time, the wiggling movement invites the muscle attachments at the hairline and around the ears to soften. This prevents tension from building up and creating blockages for the fluids. (5)

Place the gua sha tool at the center of your chin and trace along your jawline using more pressure here. If any tenderness occurs, lighten your pressure.

Now place the gua sha tool at the top of your neck. Keeping the board flat to your skin as much as possible, instead of using the edge of the tool, glide down your neck from under your ears to the top of your collarbone and repeat all the way around your neck beneath your jaw. Use extra-light pressure over your throat/larynx, or skip this area. Try not to stretch your neck upward or to the sides so that your spine remains aligned and the muscles are not engaged. Stretching your neck afterward is a wonderful addition to your routine. (6)

Acknowledge your work on the one side and then repeat the steps on to the other side.

Tip
• *Lovingly press on Joyful Sleep K 6 (see page 111) after your facial routine to invite deep, nourishing sleep, as these points will assist to calm your body and strengthen your spirit.*

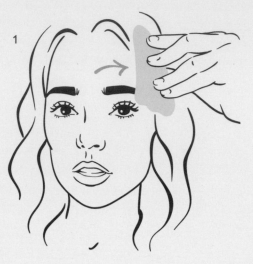

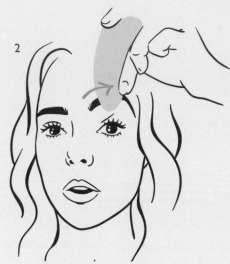

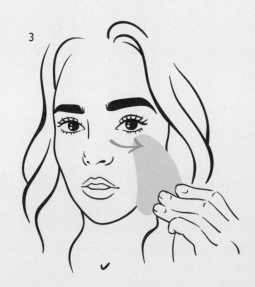

CLEARING THE CHEEKS

Often there is a little more buildup of inflammation or excess fluid in the cheeks, so a deeper massage over the lower cheeks can benefit lymph health and define your cheekbones and jawline beautifully. This is also an area where grief can be held as it represents the lungs on the facial reflexology map. Using your exhale is a powerful way to release any grief you may be holding and to also assist the lymph to release and drain down to the lymph nodes for cleansing and disposal.

BE PRESENT

Whenever I was teaching a facial workshop in a cosmopolitan city, I would incorporate this sequence, because of its relaxing and centering benefits. The audience would often reflect toward the end of the class how "grounded" and "present" they felt.

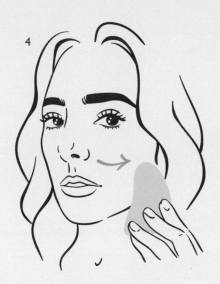

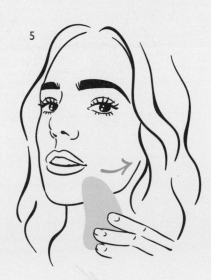

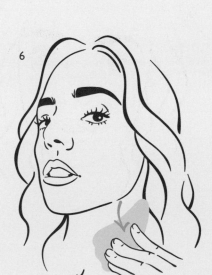

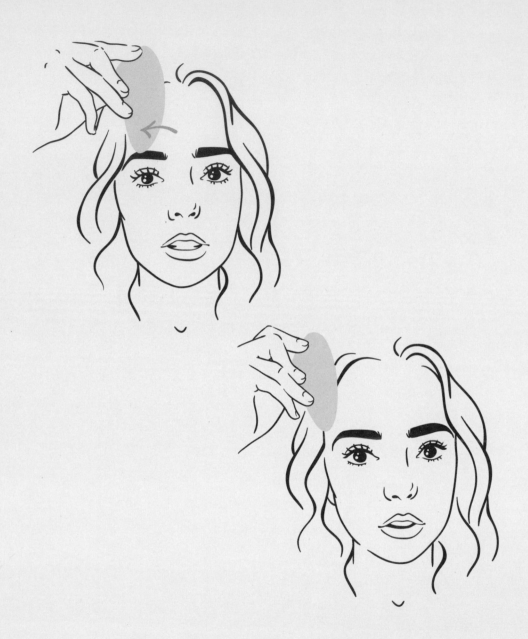

Soothe Forehead

You can think of this move as "the thought melter" or the "intuition enhancer," because it can be very relaxing and a great way to shed churning thoughts. These outward movements open up the space around the third eye as well as the liver (located between the brows on the facial map).

Lovingly massage facial oil all over your forehead.

Place the gua sha tool at the top and middle of your forehead. Sweep outward toward your hairline, connecting as much of the flat board of the tool to your skin as possible, rather than using only the edge of the tool.

Repeat this sweeping massage on the same side of your forehead from midline toward hairline until that side of your forehead has been covered.

Acknowledge your work and then repeat on the other side of your forehead.

Tips
· *Lovingly press on the Heavenly Pillar B 10 (see page 105) points located at the base of the skull on either side of your spine, to enhance the "melting of thoughts" and release anxiety, stress, burnout, and insomnia.*
· *These points have the ability to relax the whole body.*

Smooth Jaw Line

This exercise helps to release the jaw, which can have a beneficial effect on your voice, allowing you to speak more freely and clearly. Using this massage to relax these muscles and tendons at bedtime may have the ability to prevent teeth grinding and migraines caused by temporomandibular joint (TMJ) disorder.

Lovingly massage facial oil all over your chin and jawline.

Place the gua sha tool flat at the center of your chin and glide with deeper pressure over your jawline toward your earlobe. You may feel bumps of muscle tension or even hear crunchy sounds as you move over this area: these are knots of tension in the many muscles that overlap in this area.

Repeat this deeper gliding motion over your jawline three times. Then using your knuckle or the edge of the gua sha tool, find a tension knot in your jaw and massage in little circles, deepening your breath, inviting the tension to melt.

Notice the difference in how your jaw feels from one side to the other. Have a look in a mirror to see if any changes are present from one massaged side before continuing to the other.

Tip
· *Lovingly press on Wind Screen TW 17 (see page 105) located on your earlobes, to further support your jaw by relieving pain from TMJ disorder, other jaw issues, and any sore throats.*

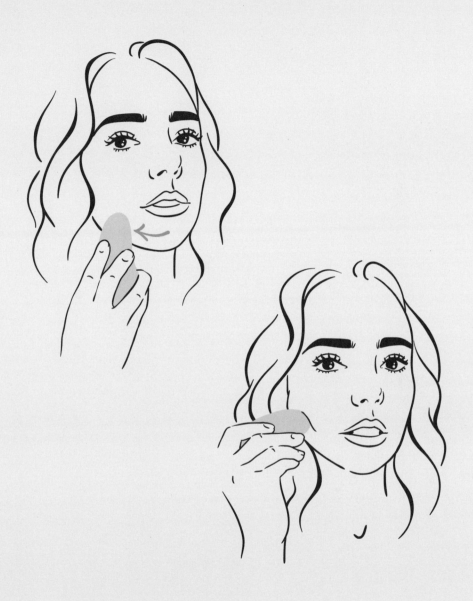

CLEARER SKIN

This point also benefits clear skin by healing or preventing acne by both releasing facial tension and supporting the immune system.

Smooth Neck and Chest

These techniques offer a great way to repattern any scrunching, rounding of the shoulders, and generally poor posture adopted during the day. The massage moves invite the heart space to open and the shoulders to soften down away from the ears and out from the center of the body.

Lovingly massage facial oil all over your neck and décolleté or chest.

Place the gua sha tool at the top of your neck beneath your earlobe and jawline. Using the flat side of the gua sha board, rather than the edge, lightly massage down to the top of your collarbone and repeat all the way around your neck. Use extra-light pressure over your throat/larynx or skip this area.

Place the gua sha tool flat to your skin at the midline of your décolleté. Glide with some pressure from your midline out toward your shoulder and armpit.

Repeat until that entire side of your chest has been massaged from just below your collarbone to the top of your breast above the nipple. Hold your skin taut with your other hand wherever feels good.

Acknowledge your work and notice any difference between the sides of your chest before moving from one to the other.

Tips
- *If you have a lot of tension in your chest, it can feel really good to use the toothed edge of a gua sha tool at a 20-degree angle or so to break up some of the adhesions or scar tissue in the muscles.*
- *Lovingly press on Elegant Mansion K 27 (see page 105) located in the soft spots right below where your collarbones come together in the middle, to elevate this technique. These points benefit the lungs, throat, and kidneys as well as resetting your own energy flow for forward and harmonized direction.*

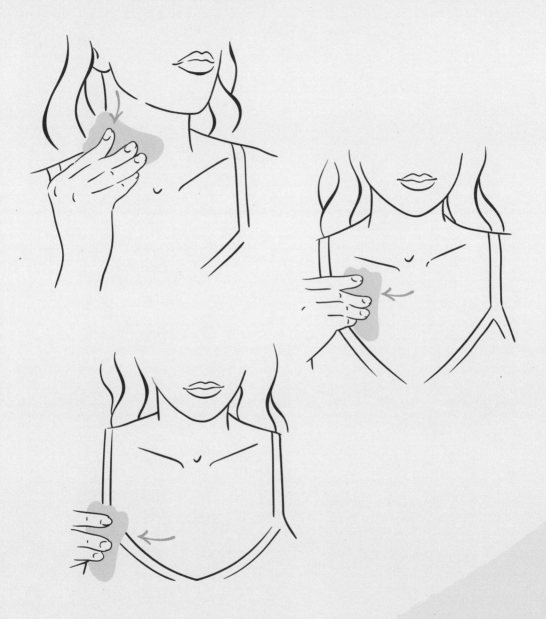

A BRAVER YOU

Repeating these massages regularly will invite you to open up and share more bravely
with others. They may also encourage you not to hide from difficult situations.

In this chapter, we combine several gua sha techniques to create sequences beneficial for three common skin complaints: blemished/acne-prone skin, dry/dehydrated skin, and pigmentation. The last sequence, the "1-Minute Facelift" (see page 138), is a quick, easy, and powerful tool if you are short on time and want instant results.

Your Bespoke Treatment Plan

CHAPTER 7

Clearing Acne/ Breakouts

Pimples and cystic acne breakouts are caused by lymph stagnation and/or a buildup in the liver. To begin your plan, drain the fluid in your neck using the Downward Neck Sweep (see page 50). Include a few optional upward strokes up the back of your neck, on either side of your spine, to release tension and open up energetic flow.

Lovingly massage facial oil all over your neck.

Place the gua sha tool at the top of your neck, just beneath your jawline, and lightly glide the tool down your neck to encourage the lymph to drain to the lymph nodes just above your collarbones. Breath deeply as you glide the gua sha tool all the way around your neck in this way. You may glide gently over your throat/larynx or you can skip that strip of your throat altogether.

Next, place the tool just under your pimple or the cluster of breakout (avoid any swollen parts of skin around an inflamed pimple, but place the tool just beneath the tender inflammation). Gently pump with the tool, as if encouraging the swelling to drop down and drain out. Repeat this gentle pumping motion about five times, stopping if any pain occurs.

Direct the fluid you have just stimulated by gliding underneath the breakout and sending the fluid toward your hairline, or along your jawline, and then sweep down your neck beneath your ear.

Repeat this draining motion three to five times unless tenderness or discomfort occurs. Sometimes nausea can come up when a lot of lymph is being drained at one time.

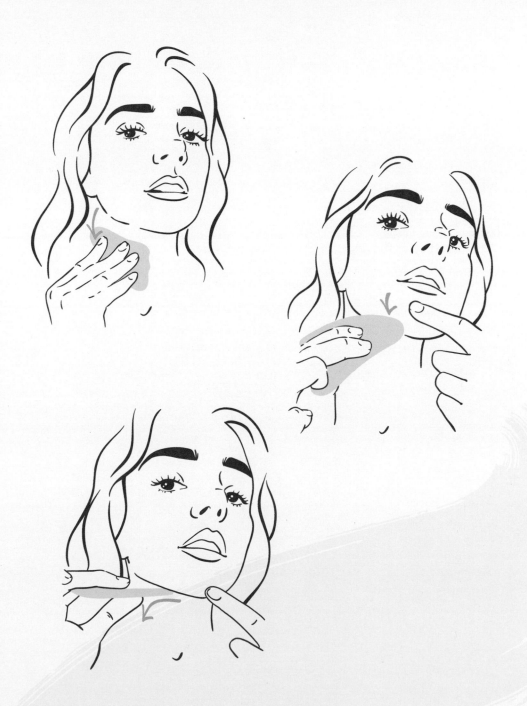

Smoothing Dry/Dehydrated Skin & Wrinkles

Dry and dehydrated skin are two different conditions. Dry skin means a lack of oils in the layers of skin tissue. Dehydrated skin refers to a lack of water in the skin's layers. Both skin issues can lead to premature or unnecessary wrinkles. Massage will restore the lipid barrier and stimulate fluid movement.

To soften your wrinkles, use a gua sha tool with a toothed edge. Hold the skin taut around the area so the tool is not dragging on the skin. Place the gua sha tool's teeth directly into the wrinkle. So, if the wrinkle is horizontal (across the forehead, at the corners of the eyes, or across the neck) place the tool's teeth horizontally into the wrinkle and then massage back and forth. This is how you break up the pattern of the wrinkle, while stimulating collagen production so this area can strengthen.

Then turn the tool vertically, and comb all along the wrinkle, up and and down, using the toothed edge. Keep the pressure very light here and the movements quite rapid. Repeat both horizontal and vertical combing several times. Stop if any pain occurs.

If the wrinkle is vertical (smile lines, lip lines, frown lines) repeat the same movements vertically and horizontally several times and holding the skin taut wherever is convenient and comfortable.

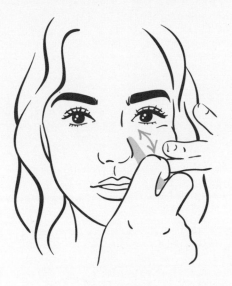

HYDRATING & NOURISHING YOUR SKIN

• Switch to an oil cleanser, which is far less drying than foam or gel cleanser.

• Encourage yourself to drink plenty of clean water (from a spring, well, or unprocessed water) from glass.

• Layer a hydrating serum underneath your facial oil or moisturizer. A serum with hyaluronic acid is very hydrating. Layering thin layers of moisture is key, especially during those dry winter months when the heat is on and the air is much more dry.

• Consult with a naturopathic doctor to see if a supplement such as flax seed oil, which has all the omegas, or an algae oil or a fish oil is right for you to nourish and hydrate your skin from within.

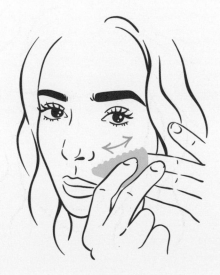

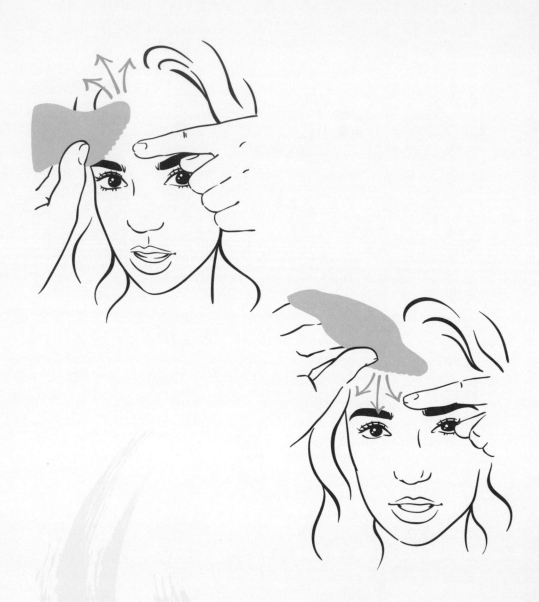

Fading Pigmentation Spots

Usually, a liver imbalance is the root cause of pigmentation irregularities. Using a gua sha tool is a great way to break up the excess buildup of proteins when there is hyperpigmentation, an excess of melanin, creating "melasma" or dark spots you would like to soften.

Lovingly apply a drop of facial oil, or more if needed, to the dark spot.

Use a gua sha tool with a toothed edge and flick from the center of the dark spot outward, as if drawing the rays on a picture of the sun. Flick outward from the middle in all directions until you have completed flicking for 360 degrees.

Keep the pressure very light. You are not trying to scrape the skin at all. Repeat this process once or twice daily. Take a "before" photo and then a "progress" photo two weeks later, to acknowledge your work.

CLEANSING YOUR LIVER

A liver cleanse and supplements that are right for your body can be co-created with the aid of a naturopathic doctor. When a liver is functioning optimally, you can receive a couple minutes of healing sun rays, without sunscreen, and not develop patches of dark spots.

1-Minute Facelift

This technique can be a favorite go-to when you are short on time. Your whole face will lift, brighten, and contour with only a few swift moves. Here is your lightening-fast pick-me-up.

Lovingly massage facial oil all over your face. Place the gua sha tool just above an eyebrow and lift up the forehead to your hairline and then continue to lift up all across your forehead.

Place the the gua sha tool on one cheek next to the bridge of your nose, and gently glide across your cheekbone toward your hairline. Repeat on the other side.

Place the gua sha tool next to your nostril and, using firmer pressure, glide underneath your cheekbones and across your lower cheeks, contouring the area and pushing out any excess inflammation or fluid toward your hairline and ears. Exhale deeply on this move. Repeat on the other side one time.

With your fingers, or with the gua sha tool, massage downward in front of your ears and then down your neck in a line under your ears. Repeat on the other side. If it feels good and you have another spare moment, repeat this move a couple more times.

Tip
• *If you have very low energy, inhale quickly through your nose, almost like "breath of fire" technique. This is a succession of tiny inhales through your nose. Then allow a long, slow exhale.*

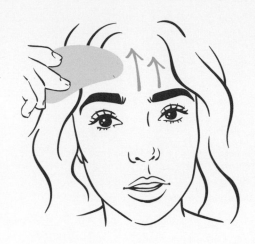

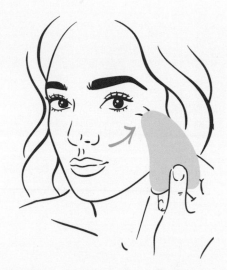

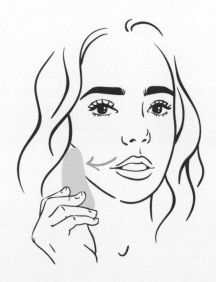

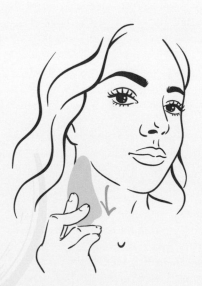

Glossary

Acupressure A form of alternative medicine in which pressing on various points on the surface of the skin stimulates or redistributes the energy within an associated organ or body system.

Collagen Matrix/Fascia Fascia is primarily made up of collagen, of which there are 28 different kinds. It lies just below the skin, connecting every organ, muscle, and joint. The nerves and lymph nodes live within this fascial/connective tissue matrix. It is also referred to as a sensory organ.

Duodenum Connecting to the stomach, the duodenum is the first part of the small intestine. It helps further digest food coming from the stomach, absorbing nutrients (vitamins, minerals, carbohydrates, fats, and proteins) and water from food so they can be used by the body.

Keloid A keloid scar is an enlarged, raised scar. They can develop after minor skin damage, from acne, or a piercing.

Lymph A watery fluid in the body that is clear to white in color. It is responsible for carrying toxins to the nearest lymph nodes, where it is cleansed before being returned to the blood.

Meridian One of several energetic pathways that run deep within the body and throughout each organ and muscle group. Acupressure points live along these meridian paths on the skin's surface and are pools of heat and electricity. Pressing on these points stimulates or redistributes the energy within the associated organ or system as well as the entire energetic meridian line that runs throughout the body.

Moxibustion The practice of burning dried mugwort herbs over acupressure points for relief. It is usually paired with acupuncture and cupping.

Reflexology The concept and associated massage practice that the entire anatomy of the body is reflected in miniature on reflex zones on the face, feet, hands, and ears.

Petechiae Red to purple bruising that appears on the skin during gua sha scraping.

Traditional Chinese Medicine (TCM) A multifaceted healing system born from alchemical Taoist texts and ancestral philosophy.

Tragus A door of cartilage that protects the entrance to the internal ear.

Yang Along with yin, one of two complementary energies considered to create a whole in traditional Chinese medicine, depicted as two black and white swirls that create a circle. Yang, the white swirl, represents masculine energies.

Yin Along with yang, one of two complementary energies considered to create a whole in traditional Chinese medicine, depicted as two black and white swirls that create a circle. Yin, the black swirl, represents feminine energies.

Resources for Further Exploration

Traditional Chinese Medicine

Maureen Tsao, M.Ac., (NCCA)
Fifth-generation acupuncturist and traditional
Chinese medicine practitioner
Graduate of Pacific Institute of Chinese
Medicine, New England School of
Acupuncture, University of San Francisco Law,
and Smith College
30 Forest Falls
Yarmouth, ME 04096
207-846-9999
https://acupuncturemaine.com/

Katya Mosely, L.Ac.
Founder and Acupuncturist of Spirit Gate
Wellness
@spiritgate.la
 www.SpiritGateLA.com
https://www.spiritgatela.com/marketplace/golden-ear-seeds

Samantha Story MS, L.Ac.
Classically trained acupuncturist with Daoist
priest and Master Acupuncturist Jeffrey Yuen
of the Jade Purity lineage
@samanthastory_
https://www.samanthastory.com/

Facial Mapping and Diagnosis

Dr. Todd Frisch
Author, "WTF? Why The Face: A Practical
Guide to Understanding Health & Personality
through Facial Diagnosis" by Dr. Todd Frisch &
Abbie Frisch Belliston
https://www.app.drtoddfrisch.com/
https://drtoddfrisch.com/
https://www.wtfwhytheface.com/

Lymph

Lisa Levitt Gainsley
Certified Manual Lymphatic Drainage
Practitioner
@thelymphaticmessage
Author, *The Book of Lymph*
https://www.thelymphaticmessage.com/online-course

Crystals and Gems

Mariah K. Lyons
Master Crystal Healer, Western Herbalist,
Reiki Master
Author, *Crystal Healing for Women*
https://linktr.ee @mariahklyons
@astara

My Reading List

Acupressure for Beginners by Bob Doto, 2019, Fair Winds Press

Acupressure's Potent Points by Michael Reed Gach, 1990, Bantam Books

The Audobon Society Pocket Guide to Familiar Rocks and Minerals of North America by Charles W. Chesterman, 1988, Knopf Publishing Group

Beauty Secrets by Dr. Ping Zhang, DOM, 2017, Nefeli Corp.

The Book of Lymph by Lisa Leavitt Gainsley, CLT, 2021, Yellow Kite

The Crystal Bible by Judy Hall, 2003, Godsfield Press

Crystal Gridwork by Kiera Fogg, 2018, Weiser Books

Crystal Muse by Heather Askinosie and Timmi Jandro, 2017, Hay House Inc.

Energy Medicine by Donna Eden with David Feinstein, PhD, 1998, Piatkus Books

Energy Medicine for Women by Donna Eden with David Feinstein, PhD, 2008, TarcherPerigee

Face Fitness by Patricia San Pedro, 2021, Chronicle Books

Face Workouts for Beginners by Nadira V. Persaud, 2020, Fair Winds Press

Five Spirits by Lorie Dechar, 2006, Lantern Books

Glow15 by Naomi Whittel, 2018, Aster

Grasping the Wind by Andrew Ellis, Nigel Wiseman, and Ken Boss, 1989, Paradigm Publications

Hildegard of Bingen's Spritual Remedies by Dr. Wighard Strehlow, 2002, Healing Arts Press

Hildegard von Bingen's Physica translated by Priscilla Throop, 1998, Healing Arts Press

The I Ching translated by C.F. Baynes, 1950, Bollingen Foundation

The Little Book of Energy Healing Techniques by Karen Frazier, 2019, Althea Press

Radical Healing by Rudolph Ballentine, MD, 1999 Himalyan Institute Press

The Seven Emotions by Claude Larre and Elisabeth Rochat de la Vallée, 1996, Monkey Press

The Subtle Body by Cyndi Dale, 2009, Sounds True, Inc.

Whole Beauty by Shiva Rose, 2018, Artisan

Why the Face by Dr. Todd Frisch and Abbie Frisch Belliston, 2019, Why the Face

Index

Acknowledgments + credits

Many hearts and hands contributed to the creation of this book and I overflow with gratitude for each and every one. Everything that comes into this world is supported by a village, seen and unseen, and I offer credit to all of us beautiful beings, including you dear one, holding this book.

Photography by Morgan Foitle, except photograph on page 7 by Kerry Crawford.

Illustrations by Olga Kamieshkova.

The tools photographed on page 26 can be credited to the following:

Rose quartz heart-shaped tool: Facial Sculptor from KORA Organics by Miranda Kerr

Jade facial roller: Province Apothecary

Wave-edged dark tool: CJB Pro Nephrite by Cecily Braden

Clear quartz tool on necklace: LINEA by Julie Civiello Polier